Eating Well
Through Cancer

Easy Recipes & Recommendations
DURING & AFTER TREATMENT

Holly Clegg & Gerald Miletello, M.D.

- **Over 200 Quick Recipes to Ease Side Effects**
- **Doc's Tips & Food Lists**
- **Nutritional Analysis**
- **Caregiver Ideas**

- **Post-Treatment Recipes**
- **Diabetic Exchanges**
- **Menus**

Photography by
David Humphreys

Dedication

*This book is dedicated to Holly's father, Jerry Berkowitz,
and everyone whose life has been touched by cancer.*

Other books by Holly Clegg
The New Holly Clegg Trim & Terrific™ Cookbook
Holly Clegg Trim & Terrific™ Home Entertaining The Easy Way
Holly Clegg Trim & Terrific™ Freezer Friendly Meals

Nutritional Analysis by Tammi Hancock, RD
Cover Design by Scott Hodgin
Photography © David Humphreys

Library of Congress Control Number: 2006924910
ISBN 10: 0-9610888-8-5
ISBN 13: 978-0-9610888-8-0

Production and Manufacturing
Favorite Recipes® Press
An imprint of

FRP.

P.O. Box 305142
Nashville, TN 37230
800-358-0560

Manufactured in the United States of America

Table of Contents

A Note on the Recipes

◆ For all recipes that call for margarine, an equal amount of butter may be substituted.

◆ The nutritional analysis provided for each recipe is based on the larger portion size listed.

◆ Although most of the recipes in this book have diabetic exchanges, not all recipes are appropriate for diabetics. Follow your doctor's recommendations.

◆ Unless otherwise stated, all eggs used should be large.

◆ Unless otherwise stated, onions and lemons should be medium size.

◆ When a recipe call for chicken broth, any type may be used, such as fat-free, low-sodium or homemade.

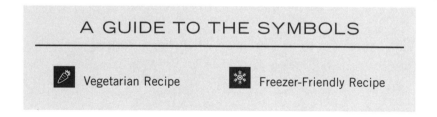

A GUIDE TO THE SYMBOLS

Vegetarian Recipe   Freezer-Friendly Recipe

Holly's Note

I enjoy eating and as author of the *Trim & Terrific* cookbook series, I strive to create recipes that are easy, healthy and delicious. Dr. Gerald Miletello, an oncologist, provided the motivation for this book. Because of my love of food, this is an opportunity for me to use my expertise in recipe development to create appropriate and best tolerated food addressing the side effects of cancer treatment. PEOPLE WITH CANCER STILL NEED TO EAT! I started researching nutrition and diet for cancer patients and found the information available to be very technical, made claims or insisted on a radical new style of eating patterns.

I believe a person should not have to eat food that does not taste good. My "no sacrifice of taste" philosophy throughout my *Trim & Terrific* cookbooks is my approach once again in creating tasty, healthy, and easy recipes. My challenge was to provide appealing recipes that ease side effects during treatment. Good nutrition and eating is essential to staying healthy and having the necessary energy.

Working with Dr. Miletello provided me with an understanding of what happens to a person having treatment. With this in mind, I tried to focus on quick recipes and include foods labeled as the "super foods" helpful in fighting cancer: cruciferous vegetables, yogurt instead of sour cream, beans, fruits, garlic, beta-carotene rich foods, fiber rich foods, beans, and fish. The recipes I created are familiar and include favorite foods but with an awareness of what a person can eat at each stage of treatment.

The *Caregiver* chapter is helpful for caregivers, family and friends. After treatment, hopefully, the joy of eating will return and the *Healthy Eating Post Treatment* chapter has recipes for a long term healthier lifestyle. *Menus* provide complete meal ideas appropriate at that time. As many recipes overlap from chapter to chapter, I think the *Recipe Cross Reference List* will prove to be a popular and invaluable source of reference.

Each recipe includes the nutritional analysis and diabetic exchange. Optional ingredients are not included in the analysis and it is based on the smaller portion serving. *Doc's Note* and my tidbits provide each recipe with valuable information. As I tested these recipes on my family, I must emphasize that anyone who enjoys a healthier approach to cooking, with or without a health problem, will also enjoy this book.

As I began my work on this cookbook, unexpectedly, it became very personal. My father was diagnosed with larynx cancer and had to undergo treatment. Eating is a necessity and I hope these recipes will make treatment a little easier with the comfort of food. My father and I love eating, and I know he will enjoy the *Healthy Eating Post Treatment* chapter for many years to come as you or your friends will! Cancer has touched everyone's life in some way and at some time. Gerald Miletello and I hope our book will touch you.

Holly Berkowitz Clegg

Dr. Miletello's Note

Cancer is an uncontrolled growth of cells that destroys the function of normal cells. Cancer can involve one organ of the body or every organ, including the blood. Once your treatment for cancer begins, you will likely notice a change in your appetite and your senses of taste and smell. The changes are secondary to normal cells being destroyed, as well as cancer cells. The goal of cancer treatment is to destroy the cancer cells and allow the good cells to flourish.

The loss of appetite, called anorexia, is one of the most common side-effects of chemotherapy. Anorexia can also result from radiation therapy, stress, anxiety, depression, and cancer itself. Trying to maintain adequate calorie intake during this time can be very difficult for the patient or caregiver who is trying to prepare food.

You have to maintain your nutrition in order to maintain your health and strength to enable you to fight the cancer. Certain foods that you once loved may no longer appeal to you. Your taste and cravings may change from day to day and hour to hour. You may develop a sore mouth and tongue or you may have trouble swallowing. Fortunately, these side-effects only last three to eight days following chemotherapy. Diarrhea and/or constipation may occur at any time during your treatments. If you are taking narcotics, constipation can become a significant problem.

Diarrhea is a condition marked by abnormally frequent bowel movements that are softer than usual. Cramping may accompany diarrhea. Diarrhea may be secondary to chemotherapy, radiation or surgery to the bowel or sometimes secondary to bowel infections from antibiotics. Milk intolerance is also a cause of diarrhea.

Neutropenia, low white blood cell count, follows most chemotherapy treatments at some time. Neutropenia normally lasts for 3–7 days. I recommend avoiding fresh fruits, vegetables, raw meat, or fish during the time your blood counts are low. As soon as your counts have returned to normal, you can return to a regular diet.

The lining or mucosa of the gastrointestinal tract, which includes the inside of the mouth and throat, is one of the most sensitive areas of the body. Many chemotherapy drugs can inflame the lining of the mouth. Many drugs can also cause ulcerations or sores to develop. This can cause difficulty maintaining your nutrition.

We hope that we can offer suggestions for food and drinks that will appeal to you, as well as suggestions for foods that will assist in managing some of the side-effects of chemotherapy. We have also included helpful hints for family and caregivers. Our last section involves healthy eating post treatment.

Although no diet has been proven to prevent cancer, health authorities agree that a properly chosen diet can reduce the risk of developing certain cancers. We also feel that a properly chosen diet can help you to fight cancer once you have developed it.

Note that any of the recipes can be tried at any time during your treatment. These recipes are all low in fat and healthy. We have also included high calorie versions of some of the recipes for whenever needed. Also, note that these foods are for everyone, not only the cancer patient. The entire family can enjoy each and every one of these dishes. We have also included diabetic exchanges since some patients are diabetic and some of the drugs we use to treat cancer will elevate your blood sugar.

Gerald Miletello, M.D.

Recipe Cross Reference List

Any of the following recipes may be high calorie by increasing your portion size.

	Day of Chemotherapy	Neutropenia	Diarrhea	Constipation	Sore Mouth or Throat	High Calorie-High Protein	Snacks and Light Meals	Caregiver	Healthy Eating Post Treatment
All Natural Laxative, page 121				✓					
Almost Better Than Sex Cake, page 257	✓	✓			✓		✓	✓	✓
Ambrosia Crumble, page 261				✓	✓		✓	✓	✓
Apple Lasagna, page 26	✓	✓		✓	✓		✓	✓	✓
Applesauce Oatmeal, page 134	✓	✓		✓	✓		✓	✓	✓
Artichoke Soup, page 60	✓			✓	✓		✓	✓	✓
Artichoke Squares, page 187		✓		✓	✓		✓	✓	✓
Asparagus and Brie Pizza, page 191				✓	✓		✓	✓	✓
Asparagus and Potato Soup, page 32	✓			✓	✓		✓	✓	✓
Avocado Soup, page 136	✓			✓	✓		✓	✓	✓
Awesome Milk Shake, page 146	✓	✓		✓	✓		✓	✓	✓
Baked Acorn Squash, page 138	✓	✓		✓	✓		✓	✓	✓
Baked Beans, page 110				✓	✓		✓	✓	✓
Baked Corn Casserole, page 111		✓		✓	✓		✓	✓	✓
Baked Fish, page 46	✓			✓	✓		✓	✓	✓
Baked French Toast, page 25	✓	✓	✓	✓	✓		✓	✓	✓
Baked Peach Delight, page 71	✓	✓		✓	✓		✓	✓	✓
Baked Topped Fish, page 247	✓	✓	✓	✓	✓		✓	✓	✓
Banana Bran Muffins, page 124				✓	✓		✓	✓	✓
Banana Bread, page 200	✓		✓	✓	✓		✓	✓	✓
Banana Cake with Cream Cheese Icing, page 258				✓	✓		✓	✓	✓
Banana Pudding, page 87	✓		✓	✓	✓		✓	✓	✓
Banana Pudding Trifle, page 50	✓			✓	✓		✓	✓	✓
Banana Puff, page 81	✓	✓	✓	✓	✓		✓	✓	✓
Banana Split Dessert, page 178	✓			✓	✓	✓	✓	✓	✓
Basic Broccoli, page 111				✓	✓		✓	✓	✓
Basic Weight Gain Shake, page 73	✓	✓		✓	✓		✓	✓	✓

Any of the following recipes may be high calorie by increasing your portion size.	Day of Chemotherapy	Neutropenia	Diarrhea	Constipation	Sore Mouth or Throat	High Calorie-High Protein	Snacks and Light Meals	Caregiver	Healthy Eating Post Treatment
Beefy Vegetable Soup, page 225				✓			✓	✓	✓
Berry French Toast, page 24	✓			✓	✓		✓	✓	✓
Black and White Bean Salad, page 108				✓			✓	✓	✓
Black Bean and Corn Salad, page 109				✓			✓	✓	✓
Blueberry Pancakes, page 23	✓			✓			✓	✓	✓
Bread Pudding Florentine, page 27	✓	✓		✓	✓		✓	✓	✓
Breakfast Casserole, page 202				✓			✓	✓	✓
Brie and Cranberry Chutney Quesadillas, page 156	✓			✓		✓	✓	✓	✓
Boiled Shrimp, page 47	✓			✓			✓	✓	✓
Burger Soup, page 158				✓		✓	✓	✓	✓
Caesar Salad, page 230				✓			✓	✓	✓
Cantaloupe Banana Smoothie, page 136	✓			✓	✓		✓	✓	✓
Carrot Soufflé, page 140	✓	✓		✓	✓		✓	✓	✓
Cauliflower Soup, page 203	✓	✓		✓	✓		✓	✓	✓
Cauliflower Supreme, page 237				✓			✓	✓	✓
Cereal Clusters, page 175				✓		✓	✓	✓	✓
Cereal Mixture, page 181	✓			✓			✓	✓	✓
Cheese Broccoli Soup, page 58		✓		✓	✓		✓	✓	✓
Cheese Quesadillas, page 193	✓	✓		✓	✓		✓	✓	✓
Cheesy Macaroni, page 40	✓	✓		✓	✓		✓	✓	✓
Cheesy Shrimp Rice Casserole, page 64	✓	✓		✓	✓		✓	✓	✓
Chess Pie, page 49	✓	✓		✓	✓		✓	✓	✓
Chicken and Black Bean Enchiladas, page 211				✓			✓	✓	✓
Chicken, Barley, and Bow-Tie Soup, page 34	✓			✓			✓	✓	✓
Chicken Diane with Wild Rice, page 43	✓			✓			✓	✓	✓
Chicken Piccata, page 66	✓	✓		✓			✓	✓	✓
Chicken Pot Pie, page 65		✓		✓			✓	✓	✓
Chicken Primavera, page 245				✓			✓	✓	✓
Chicken Salad, page 104				✓			✓	✓	✓

Any of the following recipes may be high calorie by increasing your portion size.	Day of Chemotherapy	Neutropenia	Diarrhea	Constipation	Sore Mouth or Throat	High Calorie-High Protein	Snacks and Light Meals	Caregiver	Healthy Eating Post Treatment
Chicken Scampi, page 86	✓	✓	✓				✓	✓	✓
Chicken Soup, page 33							✓	✓	✓
Chicken Tortilla Soup, page 206				✓			✓	✓	✓
Chicken with Bean Sauce, page 243				✓			✓	✓	✓
Chocolate Layered Dessert, page 219	✓						✓	✓	✓
Cinnamon Quick Bread, page 183	✓	✓			✓		✓	✓	✓
Cinnamon Rolls, page 22	✓	✓	✓				✓	✓	✓
Coffee Cake, page 196		✓					✓	✓	✓
Company Chicken, page 209							✓	✓	✓
Couscous Salad, page 226	✓			✓			✓	✓	✓
Crabmeat Egg Casserole, page 30	✓						✓	✓	✓
Cream Cheese Bread Pudding, page 145	✓	✓			✓		✓	✓	✓
Cream of Spinach and Brie Soup, page 137					✓		✓	✓	✓
Cream of Spinach Soup, page 205				✓	✓		✓	✓	✓
Creamed Double Potatoes, page 141				✓	✓		✓	✓	✓
Creamy Squash Casserole, page 82			✓				✓	✓	✓
Curried Rice and Sweet Potatoes, page 235				✓			✓	✓	✓
Easy Banana Bread, page 80	✓	✓	✓		✓		✓	✓	✓
Easy Beef Enchiladas, page 164				✓		✓	✓	✓	✓
Easy Brisket, page 170				✓		✓	✓	✓	✓
Easy Broccoli Potato Bake, page 236							✓	✓	✓
Easy Chili, page 159					✓	✓	✓	✓	✓
Easy Crab Soup, page 61				✓			✓	✓	✓
Easy Cranberry Yam Bread, page 126	✓	✓		✓			✓	✓	✓
Egg Noodle Casserole, page 29		✓					✓	✓	✓
Egg Soufflé, page 28	✓				✓		✓	✓	✓
Eggplant Parmesan, page 241	✓				✓		✓	✓	✓
Fabulous Fruit Dip, page 177				✓		✓	✓	✓	✓
Fortified Milk, page 153	✓	✓		✓	✓	✓	✓	✓	✓

Any of the following recipes may be high calorie by increasing your portion size.	Day of Chemotherapy	Neutropenia	Diarrhea	Constipation	Sore Mouth or Throat	High Calorie-High Protein	Snacks and Light Meals	Caregiver	Healthy Eating Post Treatment
Fresh Fruit Dip, page 185	✓						✓	✓	✓
Fresh Tomato and Cheese Pizza, page 190							✓	✓	✓
Fried Rice Stir-Fry, page 234				✓			✓	✓	✓
Fruity Couscous Salad, page 35	✓			✓			✓	✓	✓
German Chocolate Angel Pie, page 144	✓	✓			✓		✓	✓	✓
Ginger Chicken and Black Beans, page 166					✓	✓	✓	✓	✓
Glazed Bananas, page 88	✓		✓				✓	✓	✓
Granola, page 92				✓			✓	✓	✓
Grilled Pork Tenderloin, page 254			✓				✓	✓	✓
Ham and Cheese Grits Quiche, page 142	✓	✓			✓		✓	✓	✓
Heavenly Yam Delight, page 69		✓					✓	✓	✓
Herb Baked Salmon, page 250							✓	✓	✓
Herbed Shrimp, page 247							✓	✓	✓
Honey Bran Prune Muffins, page 124				✓			✓	✓	✓
Hot Cocoa Drink Supplement, page 74	✓	✓			✓		✓	✓	✓
Hot Fruit Compote, page 68	✓	✓		✓	✓		✓	✓	✓
Indoor Barbecue Roasted Salmon, page 169				✓		✓	✓	✓	✓
Italian Chicken, page 44	✓						✓	✓	✓
Italian Pasta Salad, page 188							✓	✓	✓
Italian Spinach Pie, page 194				✓			✓	✓	✓
Italian-Style Pot Roast, page 253				✓			✓	✓	✓
Italian Veal Supreme, page 256				✓			✓	✓	✓
Jumbo Stuffed Shells, page 214				✓			✓	✓	✓
Lemon Angel Food Cake, page 51	✓	✓			✓		✓	✓	✓
Lemon Berry Bread, 125	✓			✓			✓	✓	✓
Lemon Chicken with Feta, page 167	✓		✓			✓	✓	✓	✓
Linguine Florentine, page 62		✓			✓		✓	✓	✓
Loaded Potatoes, page 63	✓	✓			✓		✓	✓	✓
Mandarin Chicken Salad, page 105				✓			✓	✓	✓

Any of the following recipes may be high calorie by increasing your portion size.	Day of Chemotherapy	Neutropenia	Diarrhea	Constipation	Sore Mouth or Throat	High Calorie-High Protein	Snacks and Light Meals	Caregiver	Healthy Eating Post Treatment
Manicotti, page 208				✓	✓		✓	✓	✓
Mashed Potatoes, page 161	✓			✓	✓	✓	✓	✓	✓
Meat Loaf, page 120				✓			✓	✓	✓
Meaty Cabbage Casserole, page 252				✓			✓	✓	✓
Melon Soup, page 132	✓				✓		✓	✓	✓
Mexican Chicken Casserole, page 210				✓			✓	✓	✓
Minestrone, page 101				✓			✓	✓	✓
Mini Cheese Pizzas, page 189	✓	✓					✓	✓	✓
Mocha Cappuccino Pudding Pie, page 70		✓			✓		✓	✓	✓
Mocha Meringue Mounds, page 198	✓	✓	✓		✓		✓	✓	✓
Mock Chocolate Éclair, page 52	✓	✓			✓		✓	✓	✓
Mushroom Barley Soup, page 97				✓			✓	✓	✓
No Bake Cookies, page 197							✓	✓	✓
Noodle Pudding, page 139		✓			✓		✓	✓	✓
Oatmeal Chocolate Cake, page 127	✓			✓			✓	✓	✓
Oatmeal Pancakes, page 224	✓	✓		✓	✓		✓	✓	✓
Orzo Asparagus Toss, page 41	✓			✓			✓	✓	✓
Oven Fried Parmesan Chicken, page 84	✓	✓	✓				✓	✓	✓
Paella Salad, page 227				✓			✓	✓	✓
Pasta Salad, page 215				✓			✓	✓	✓
Pasta Toss, page 82			✓				✓	✓	✓
Peach Crumble, page 128	✓			✓	✓		✓	✓	✓
Peach Smoothie, page 72	✓	✓			✓		✓	✓	✓
Peach Soup, page 31	✓						✓	✓	✓
Peach Weight Gain Shake, page 72	✓	✓			✓		✓	✓	✓
Peanut Butter-Banana Pie, page 260					✓		✓	✓	✓
Peanut Butter Snack Spread, page 176	✓			✓	✓	✓	✓	✓	✓
Perfect Pasta, page 38	✓	✓			✓		✓	✓	✓
Pesto Pasta, page 238							✓	✓	✓

Any of the following recipes may be high calorie by increasing your portion size.	Day of Chemotherapy	Neutropenia	Diarrhea	Constipation	Sore Mouth or Throat	High Calorie-High Protein	Snacks and Light Meals	Caregiver	Healthy Eating Post Treatment
Pork Medallions, page 172			✓			✓	✓	✓	✓
Potato Pizza, page 39	✓						✓	✓	✓
Pretzel Strawberry Gelatin, page 217	✓						✓	✓	✓
Pumpkin Soup, page 57	✓	✓			✓		✓	✓	✓
Quick and Easy Corn and Shrimp Soup, page 204							✓	✓	✓
Quick Black Bean Soup, page 160				✓		✓	✓	✓	✓
Quick Cheese Grits, page 56	✓	✓	✓		✓		✓	✓	✓
Quick Cheesy Potato Soup, page 203					✓		✓	✓	✓
Quick Chicken and Dumplings, page 45	✓	✓			✓		✓	✓	✓
Quick Chicken Pasta, page 85			✓				✓	✓	✓
Quick Herb Chicken, page 244	✓		✓				✓	✓	✓
Quick Loaded Chicken Enchiladas, page 165				✓		✓	✓	✓	✓
Quick Shrimp Sauté, page 143					✓		✓	✓	✓
Quick Veggie Soup, page 98				✓			✓	✓	✓
Raspberry Spinach Salad, page 231				✓			✓	✓	✓
Rice Taco Salad, page 207							✓	✓	✓
Roasted Turkey Breast, page 83	✓	✓	✓				✓	✓	✓
Salmon Patties with Horseradish Caper Sauce, page 248							✓	✓	✓
Savory Lamb Chops, page 255							✓	✓	✓
Seafood and Wild Rice Casserole, page 212				✓			✓	✓	✓
Seven-Layer Salad, page 228							✓	✓	✓
Shrimp and Cheese Grits, page 154	✓			✓		✓	✓	✓	✓
Shrimp and Squash Scampi, page 119				✓			✓	✓	✓
Shrimp and Wild Rice Salad, page 106				✓			✓	✓	✓
Shrimp, Peppers, and Cheese Grits, page 246							✓	✓	✓
Shrimp Rice Casserole, page 216							✓	✓	✓
Shrimp Scampi with White Beans, page 168				✓		✓	✓	✓	✓
Simple Vichyssoise, page 132					✓		✓	✓	✓
Simply Delicious Chicken, page 42	✓						✓	✓	✓

Any of the following recipes may be high calorie by increasing your portion size.	Day of Chemotherapy	Neutropenia	Diarrhea	Constipation	Sore Mouth or Throat	High Calorie-High Protein	Snacks and Light Meals	Caregiver	Healthy Eating Post Treatment
Simply Salmon Pasta, page 249							✓	✓	✓
Smothered Round Steak, page 171				✓		✓	✓	✓	✓
Snack Mix, page 182				✓			✓	✓	✓
Southwestern Chicken with Salsa, page 242							✓	✓	✓
Southwestern Egg Wraps, page 155				✓		✓	✓	✓	✓
Southwestern Pasta, page 118				✓			✓	✓	✓
Southwestern Stuffed Potatoes, page 195				✓			✓	✓	✓
Spinach and Black Bean Enchiladas, page 163				✓		✓	✓	✓	✓
Spinach and Cheese Tortilla Pizza, page 192							✓	✓	✓
Spinach Dip, page 184	✓	✓			✓		✓	✓	✓
Spinach Layered Dish, page 201	✓			✓			✓	✓	✓
Spinach Rice with Feta, page 233				✓			✓	✓	✓
Split Pea and Pasta Soup, 99	✓			✓			✓	✓	✓
Squash and Tomato Casserole, 239				✓			✓	✓	✓
Squash Bisque, page 100				✓			✓	✓	✓
Strawberry Angel Food Cake, page 259	✓						✓	✓	✓
Strawberry Fruit Dip, page 185	✓						✓	✓	✓
Strawberry Raspberry Soup, page 93	✓			✓			✓	✓	✓
Strawberry Salsa, page 186				✓			✓	✓	✓
Strawberry Slush, page 181				✓					
Strawberry Soup, page 31	✓			✓			✓	✓	✓
Strawberry Weight Gain Shake, page 146	✓			✓			✓	✓	✓
Sweet and Sour Broccoli Salad, page 229				✓			✓	✓	✓
Sweet Potato and Apple Soup, page 102				✓	✓		✓	✓	✓
Sweet Potato, Apple, and Walnut Muffins, page 123				✓			✓	✓	✓
Sweet Potato Bisque, page 157	✓	✓		✓	✓	✓	✓	✓	✓
Sweet Potato Pancakes with Apple Walnut Topping, page 94				✓			✓	✓	✓
Sweet Poato Pound Cake, 220							✓	✓	✓
Sweet Potato Shake, 136				✓	✓		✓	✓	✓

Any of the following recipes may be high calorie by increasing your portion size.	Day of Chemotherapy	Neutropenia	Diarrhea	Constipation	Sore Mouth or Throat	High Calorie-High Protein	Snacks and Light Meals	Caregiver	Healthy Eating Post Treatment
Tasty Brown Rice, page 112				✓			✓	✓	✓
Tasty Tropical Smoothie, page 153	✓			✓		✓	✓	✓	✓
Tropical Green Salad, page 232				✓			✓	✓	✓
Tropical Pizza, page 218				✓			✓	✓	✓
Tropical Salsa, 95				✓			✓	✓	✓
Tuna Pasta Salad, 107				✓			✓	✓	✓
Tuna Salad, 37	✓			✓			✓	✓	✓
Tuna Steaks with Horseradish Sauce, page 251							✓	✓	✓
Turkey Jambalaya, page 213				✓			✓	✓	✓
Two-Potato Bisque, page 59	✓	✓			✓		✓	✓	✓
Veal and Broccoli with Tomato Vinaigrette, page 173				✓		✓	✓	✓	✓
Vegetable au Gratin, page 162						✓	✓	✓	✓
Vegetable Lasagna, page 117				✓			✓	✓	✓
Veggie Angel Hair, page 114				✓			✓	✓	✓
Very Good Veal, page 67		✓					✓	✓	✓
Waldorf Pasta Salad, page 36	✓			✓			✓	✓	✓
Waldorf Salad, 103				✓			✓	✓	✓
Watermelon Slush, page 135	✓				✓		✓	✓	✓
Weight Gain Pancakes, page 133		✓			✓		✓	✓	✓
White Bean and Tortellini Soup, page 96				✓			✓	✓	✓
Wild Rice and Barley Pilaf, page 113				✓			✓	✓	✓
Yam Biscuits, page 48	✓	✓			✓		✓	✓	✓
Yam Cornbread Stuffing, 240				✓			✓	✓	✓
Yam Veggie Wraps, 116				✓			✓	✓	✓
Ziti with Broccoli and White Beans Topped with Tuna, page 174				✓		✓	✓	✓	✓
Zucchini Oatmeal-Raisin Muffins, 122				✓			✓	✓	✓

Day of Chemotherapy
AND FOLLOWING TREATMENT

- ✦ What should I eat prior to my treatment?
- ✦ Is there a certain time of day that is better for eating?
- ✦ I only like two foods!
- ✦ I cannot eat, but I can drink!
- ✦ Nothing tastes good!
- ✦ How do I overcome weight loss?
- ✦ How do I prepare my pantry?

Not all treatments will cause nausea, vomiting or loss of appetite. The acute side effects, such as nausea, are caused by the destruction of rapidly dividing cells lining the gastrointestinal tract. This is one of the primary causes for the loss of appetite, nausea, vomiting and sore mouth.

I recommend a low fat, light meal prior to your treatment, including foods such as cereal, toast, oatmeal, grits, fruit cocktail, peach or pear nectar. Twenty-four hours following your treatment I would try liquids, soups, puddings or sandwiches. Try to avoid high fat, fried or greasy foods for the first twenty-four to forty-eight hours following treatment. If you find that only two foods appeal to you, then there is nothing wrong with eating those foods until you feel like expanding your diet. Water is essential. I recommend eight to ten glasses of water per day. Supplements such as Boost are excellent choices if you only feel like drinking.

You may experience a sore or dry mouth as well as a total loss of appetite. This may require a little creativity on you part to keep your nutritional status on the positive side. You may find it impossible to eat three large meals per day. This is the first time in your life that someone is going to recommend to you that you eat snacks daily. Six small meals instead of three large meals will increase your caloric intake. Remember hydration is of utmost importance. Keep a glass of liquid available at all times. (Water with a slice of lemon, apple juice, carrot juice, cranberry juice etc.) Do not forget your mouth care protocol. This really will keep your mouth refreshed and decrease ulcer formation.

Mix one teaspoon of salt with one teaspoon of baking soda in a quart of water. Rinse and spit after each meal or at least four times per day. Mix fresh each morning using tap water.

Remember your mouth will get better. The soreness normally clears within a few days. Food is medicine. You have to eat to get through these treatments and back to normal. Rinsing with

Ulcerease, Viscous Xylocaine, or Cephacol lozenges may soothe your mouth before a meal. Avoid any food that may irritate your mouth. This would include oranges, lemons, tomato sauces, crackers and alcohol. Avoid hot or extremely cold foods since they tend to irritate your mouth.

Foods at room temperature or slightly cool foods are much more soothing. Try cutting your food into small pieces, cook food until tender or even try pureeing food with a food processor. Drinking with a straw will sometimes help liquids go down easier.

Day of Chemotherapy and Following Treatment Tips
+ Eat smaller portions more frequently. Drink fluids between meals instead of with food.
+ Eat by the clock at regularly scheduled times. Your appetite signal may not be intact.
+ Eat between meals with high-protein diet supplements, milkshakes, puddings, or nutritional energy drink supplement.
+ Add cream or butter to soups, cooked cereals, and vegetables to increase calories. Add gravies and sauces to vegetables, meat, poultry and fish until weight loss is no longer a problem.
+ Add extra protein to your diet by using fortified milk, peanut butter, cheese and chopped hard boiled eggs.
+ Try things to enhance smell, appearance, and texture of food. Be creative with desserts.
+ Choose foods you like as long as you do not have dietary restrictions.
+ Exercise approximately 30 minutes before meals, to try to stimulate your appetite.
+ Try to make mealtimes pleasant by setting an attractive table and by eating with family or friends.
+ Plan menus in advance. Have some food frozen and ready to heat and serve.

If you experience changes in taste, hopefully these suggestions will help:
+ Cancer and its treatments can cause changes in your senses of taste and smell. If you are having this problem, try foods or beverages that are different from ones you usually eat. Also, keep your mouth clean by rinsing and brushing, which in turn may improve the taste of foods.
+ Season foods with tart flavors such as lemon wedges, lemonade, citrus fruits, vinegar, and pickled foods. (If you have a sore mouth or throat, do not use this tip.)

- Tart candies, peppermint or lemon drops may reduce the sensations of bitter or sour taste. Try choosing sugarless kinds. Try drinking lemonade.
- If you experience that "metallic" taste in meat, try marinating meat in a reduced sodium soy sauce or fat free Italian dressing to intensify the flavor. If red meat doesn't work, try eating chicken, seafood or beans for protein.
- Add strongly flavored juices or relishes.
- Add extra seasonings to give the food more flavor such as onion, garlic, chili powder, basil, oregano, rosemary, tarragon, barbecue sauce, mustard, ketchup, or mint. The rule of thumb is to add a little at a time to see if you can perk up those taste buds.
- Try eating foods that don't have strong odors.
- Eat foods at room temperature. This can decrease the food tastes and smells.
- Increase the sugar in foods to increase their pleasant tastes and decrease salty, bitter, or acid tastes.
- Rinse your mouth with tea, ginger ale, salted water, or water with baking soda before eating to help clear your taste buds.
- Fresh vegetables may be more appealing than canned or frozen ones.
- Use plastic utensils if you're bothered by a bitter or metallic taste.
- Maybe foods that you didn't enjoy in the past will be palate pleasing now. This is a great time to try new foods.
- Sucking on a thin slice of dill pickle, prior to meals, will sometimes stimulate your taste buds.

Changes in Food's Flavor

Cancer often affects the taste buds, commonly reducing the ability to taste sweetness. This changes the flavor of sweets, desserts, fruits and vegetables.

- Use extra sugar with many desserts to improve the taste or to provide its accustomed taste. A teaspoon of sugar added to cooking water or glazing vegetables such as may help improve vegetable flavors.
- Some people experience an unusual dislike for certain foods, flavors, or odors. This develops when unpleasant symptoms are tied to a food recently eaten.

- ✦ Save your favorite foods for times when you feel well. Try not to eat one to two hours before treatment or therapy. If you no longer enjoy beef or pork, you may find chicken, fish, eggs, milk products or legumes more appealing.
- ✦ Marinate meats or cook them with sauces or tomatoes to help improve the flavor. Meats that are cold or at room temperature may be more palatable.
- ✦ A third potential taste change is an increased liking for tart flavors. Adding lemon juice to foods may make them taste better. A cancer patient may enjoy grapefruit, cranberry, or other tart juices.

Stocking the Pantry

Preparation and organization are the two key words. The goal of a well stocked pantry should be to have enough food stored to prepare satisfying meals to limit the trips to the grocery store. Be sure to consider, along with the pantry, the refrigerator and freezer.

Begin by including items that you know you like and use most often. Gradually add to your herb and spice inventory. Remember, at this time in your life, your tastes might be slightly different and the pantry may need to include items that appeal to you now. A variety of pasta, rice, and beans and grains may be included, however, if you don't have the exact kind called for in a recipe, just substitute another type you have in the pantry. Canned broths, canned tomatoes, and olive oil are staple items that will be used often.

For the freezer, purchase skinless boneless chicken breasts, pork tenderloins, and ground sirloin. Whenever you are buying meat, always look for the leanest cuts which have a round or sirloin in their name. Then trim any visible fat before preparing. Try making individual hamburger patties wrapped in plastic wrap for a quick pull out. They can be used for sandwiches or defrosted for a recipe. Frozen yogurts are great for that ice cream urge and bags of frozen fruit will be useful. When preparing soups, double the recipe and freeze in zip top bags. Get rid of the air bubbles and they stack easily in the freezer. Convenience items such as frozen veggies are a must and can include spinach, broccoli or your favorites.

For the refrigerator, purchase low fat or fat free dairy products. If you need extra calories, there will be other opportunities as you don't need extra saturated fat. Eggs, margarine, and cheese are also dairy staples.

REFRIGERATOR STAPLES

- Refrigerated biscuits
- Butter or margarine
- Egg
- Cheese (varieties or reduced fat)
- Fruit
- Onion (yellow and green)
- Garlic (chopped in jar, fresh)
- Green pepper
- Horseradish
- Lemon and lime juice
- Mixed greens
- Skim milk
- Sour cream (fat free or light)
- Fresh vegetables
- Yogurt (fat free or light)

PANTRY STAPLES

- Barley
- Beans (canned)
- Bread (whole wheat or white)
- Bread crumbs (Italian or plain)
- Broth (canned, cubes, granules)
- Bulgur
- Couscous
- Evaporated skimmed milk
- Green chilies (diced)
- Oils (canola, peanut, olive)
- Pasta (assorted shapes and flavors)
- Pizza crusts, focaccia bread, Boboli
- Rice (white, brown, quick cooking)
- Salsas, flavored salsas
- Sauces, marinades (ready-made)
- Tomatoes, paste, sauce (all types canned)
- Tuna, salmon, chicken (canned)
- Vinegar (balsamic, rice, wine)

BAKING STAPLES

- Baking powder
- Baking soda
- Cake mixes (chocolate, yellow, white)
- Semi-sweet chocolate chips
- Canola oil
- Cocoa
- Cornstarch
- Dried Fruit
- Evaporated skimmed milk
- Flour (all purpose, self-rising, whole wheat)
- Instant pudding
- Nonstick cooking spray

- Nuts
- Oatmeal
- Sugar (confectioners' granulated, brown, artificial sweetener)
- Sweetened condensed milk (fat free or reduced fat)
- Extracts (vanilla, almond, butter, coconut)

CONDIMENT STAPLES

- Capers
- Hot sauce
- Honey
- Ketchup
- Mayonnaise (light or low fat)
- Mustard (Dijon or yellow)
- Roasted red peppers (bottled)
- Pasta sauces (jars)
- Salad dressing (fat free or reduced fat)
- Salsa
- Soy sauce (reduced sodium)
- Vinegar (balsamic, cider, distilled)
- Worcestershire sauce

SPICE PANTRY STAPLES

- Basil leaves
- Bay leaves

- Chili powder
- Cilantro
- Cinnamon (ground)
- Cumin (ground)
- Curry
- Dill weed
- Garlic powder
- Ginger (ground)
- Nutmeg
- Oregano leaves
- Paprika
- Parsley flakes (dried)
- Pepper (black, coarsely ground, red pepper flakes)

- Rosemary leaves
- Tarragon leaves
- Thyme leaves

CANNED GOODS
- Beans (assorted)
- Black olives
- Broth (beef, chicken, vegetable)
- Corn
- Creamed soups (reduced fat)
- Green chilies (diced)
- Tomatoes (diced, sauce)

- Diced tomatoes and green chilies
- Tuna and salmon

FROZEN PANTRY STAPLES
- Chicken breasts
- Fish
- Frozen veggies (i.e. spinach, corn)
- Pork tenders
- Shrimp
- Sirloin (ground, roast)
- Turkey breast
- Yogurt or ice cream (reduced fat or fat free)

Tips to Ease At-Home Cooking
- Wash and dry lettuce and seal in plastic containers or a greens bag for easy use.
- Wash, cut up and store veggies to have ready for snacks or use in recipes.
- Raid the salad bar for cut up veggies for recipes or for ready to eat products.
- Shred cheese and store in zip top bags or buy shredded cheese.
- When chopping onion or garlic, chop more than needed and store in zip top bags in the freezer for later use.
- Double recipes to freeze some for a later date or freeze extra.

Shopping List for the Day of Chemotherapy
- Bananas
- Butter
- Canned chicken broth
- Cheese
- Skinless boneless chicken
- Cream of Wheat
- Eggs

- Grits
- Instant puddings, gelatins
- Pasta
- Potatoes
- Roasted Turkey
- Rice
- Toast, crackers or pretzels

Menus

Foods to eat on the day of chemotherapy and following treatment.

Morning of Chemotherapy

Eggs, Cereal, Juice
Oatmeal, Grits, Fruit
Tea, Coffee, Sports Drink

Evening of Chemotherapy

Soup, Cheese Toast, Water, Sports Drink
Pudding, Raisins, Noodles with Cheese
Peanut Butter and Jelly Sandwich
Ham and Cheese Sandwich
Remember 6 to 8 cups of fluid per day
Nutritional Supplement Shake

Morning Following Chemotherapy

Tea, Toast
Fresh Fruit
Yogurt
Instant Breakfast

Lunch 24 Hours Past Chemotherapy

Chicken, Barley, and Bow-Tie Soup   34
Tuna Salad   37
Water

Dinner 24 Hours Past Chemotherapy

Perfect Pasta   38
Cheesy Macaroni   40
Simply Delicious Chicken   42
Yam Biscuits   48
Water

Cinnamon Rolls

When you have the urge for a wonderful cinnamon roll, make this quick recipe using canned biscuits and pantry ingredients.

MAKES 10 ROLLS

1 (10-biscuit) can refrigerated biscuits or
   whole wheat biscuits
4 tablespoons margarine, softened
2 tablespoons sugar
1 teaspoon ground cinnamon
1/4 cup raisins, optional
1/4 cup chopped pecans, optional

Preheat oven to 425 degrees. Flatten each biscuit with your hand or a rolling pin. Spread each biscuit with margarine. In a small bowl, combine the sugar and cinnamon together. Sprinkle cinnamon mixture on top of margarine; sprinkle with raisin and pecans, if desired. Roll up each biscuit from one side to the other. On an ungreased 15×10×1-inch baking sheet, arrange each biscuit roll to form a circle touching one end of the roll to the other. Bake for 8 to 10 minutes.

Nutritional information per serving
Calories 101, Protein (g) 1, Carbohydrate (g) 12, Fat (g) 5, Cal. from Fat (%) 46, Saturated Fat (g) 1, Dietary Fiber (g) 0, Cholesterol (mg) 0, Sodium (mg) 233, Diabetic Exchanges: 1 starch, 1 fat

DOC'S NOTES:

Great dessert or breakfast accompaniment.

Blueberry Pancakes 🥕 ❄️

These pancakes are so good you won't need much syrup or margarine.

MAKES 8 TO 10 PANCAKES

1 cup buttermilk

4 large egg whites

2 tablespoons sugar

1½ tablespoons canola oil

1 cup all-purpose flour

1 teaspoon baking powder

½ teaspoon baking soda

1 cup blueberries, fresh or frozen (thawed)

In a large mixing bowl, beat together the buttermilk, egg whites, sugar, and oil. In another mixing bowl, combine together the flour, baking powder, and baking soda. Add the flour mixture to the buttermilk mixture, blending well. Stir the blueberries in gently. Coat a nonstick skillet with nonstick cooking spray and heat over medium heat. Pour the batter in 1/4-cup portions onto the skillet and cook until brown on both sides and firm to touch, about 3 minutes per side.

Nutritional information per serving

Calories 98, Protein (g) 4, Carbohydrate (g) 16, Fat (g) 2, Cal. from Fat (%) 22, Saturated Fat (g) 0, Dietary Fiber (g) 1, Cholesterol (mg) 1, Sodium (mg) 160, Diabetic Exchanges: 1 starch

DOC'S NOTES:

You can substitute vanilla nutritional energy drink supplement for the buttermilk. Blueberries are a good source of phyto chemicals which may help prevent cancer.

Berry French Toast ✦

Use whatever fresh berries you can find or pull them out of the freezer and enjoy this incredible version of French toast. Try using whole grain bread.

MAKES 8 SERVINGS

5 cups mixed berries (strawberries and
   blueberries, etc.)

1/4 cup sugar plus 1 tablespoon sugar, divided

1 teaspoon ground cinnamon

I large egg

4 large egg whites, beaten

1 cup skim milk

1 teaspoon vanilla extract

1 (16-ounce) loaf French bread,
   sliced in 1-inch slices

Preheat oven to 350 degrees. In an oblong 2-quart casserole, put berries, 1/4 cup sugar, and cinnamon. In a large bowl combine egg, egg whites, milk, and vanilla. Add bread and soak for 5 minutes turning half way through. Arrange bread in one layer over berries. Sprinkle with remaining sugar. Bake for 25 to 30 minutes or until bread is golden. Serve with berry juice and berries.

Nutritional information per serving

Calories 253, Protein (g) 9, Carbohydrate (g) 48,
Fat (g) 3, Cal. from Fat (%) 10, Saturated Fat (g) 1,
Dietary Fiber (g) 4, Cholesterol (mg) 27, Sodium (mg) 396,
Diabetic Exchanges: 0.5 very lean meat, 2 starch, 1 fruit

DOC'S NOTES:

Breakfast foods can be eaten in the morning or evening. The berries provide a good source of Vitamin C and potassium, and fiber is in relatively good supply, too.

Baked French Toast 🥕

The orange juice and maple syrup make this a light, not-too-sweet dish.

MAKES 8 SERVING

3 tablespoons margarine, melted
1/3 cup maple syrup
1 teaspoon ground cinnamon
1 large egg
4 large egg whites
1 cup orange juice
8 slices white or whole wheat bread

Preheat oven to 375 degrees. Combine the margarine and syrup together in a 13×9×2-inch baking pan and sprinkle with the cinnamon. In a mixing bowl, beat together the egg, egg whites, and orange juice. Dip the bread into the egg mixture and arrange in single layer in the baking pan. Bake for 20 to 25 minutes, or until the bread is light brown.

Nutritional information per serving

Calories 185, Protein (g) 5, Carbohydrate (g) 28, Fat (g) 6, Cal. from Fat (%) 29, Saturated Fat (g) 1, Dietary Fiber (g) 1, Cholesterol (mg) 27, Sodium (mg) 248, Diabetic Exchanges: 1 starch, 0.5 fruit, 0.5 other carb., 1 fat

DOC'S NOTES:

Beware of the orange juice if your mouth is sore.

Apple Lasagna 🥕 ❄️

Apples and pasta pair up for this unusual combo. Wonderful for breakfast, a light dinner, or even as a side.

MAKES 10 TO 12 SERVINGS

8 lasagna noodles
2 (21-ounce) cans apple pie filling
1 (15-ounce) container part skim ricotta cheese
2 large egg whites
1 teaspoon almond extract
1/4 cup sugar
1/3 cup all-purpose flour
1 teaspoon ground cinnamon
3 tablespoons margarine
1/3 cup light brown sugar
1/3 cup old-fashioned oatmeal
1/2 teaspoon vanilla extract

Preheat oven to 350 degrees. Prepare lasagna noodles according to package directions; drain. Spread one can apple pie filling in a 13×9×2-inch pan coated with nonstick cooking spray, slicing any extra-thick apples. Cover apples with four lasagna noodles. In a bowl, mix together ricotta cheese, egg whites, almond extract, and sugar. Spread evenly over lasagna noodles and top with the remaining four lasagna noodles. Spoon remaining can of apple pie filling over lasagna. In a small bowl, crumble together flour, cinnamon, margarine, brown sugar, oatmeal, and vanilla. Sprinkle over apple filling. Bake for 45 minutes. Let stand 15 minutes.

Nutritional information per serving

Calories 292, Protein (g) 7, Carbohydrate (g) 53, Fat (g) 6, Cal. from Fat (%) 19, Saturated Fat (g) 2, Dietary Fiber (g) 2, Cholesterol (mg) 11, Sodium (mg) 133, Diabetic Exchanges: 0.5 very lean meat, 1 starch, 2 fruit, 0.5 other carb., 1 fat

DOC'S NOTES:

This can also serve as a dessert or midday snack. The apples are a good source of fiber.

Bread Pudding Florentine 🥕 ❄️

Adjust the mushrooms and onions to your taste buds. Here's a great make-ahead dish. Pop in a cold oven if using a glass dish when baking. Breakfast type foods are enjoyed all times of day.

MAKES 10 TO 12 SERVINGS

5 large eggs

4 large egg whites

3 cups skim milk

1/4 cup Dijon mustard

Salt and pepper to taste

1 (16-ounce) loaf day-old French bread, cut into 16 slices, divided

1/2 pound mushrooms, sliced

1 teaspoon minced garlic

1 onion, chopped

2 (10-ounce) boxes frozen chopped spinach, thawed and squeezed dry

1 tablespoon all-purpose flour

Salt and pepper to taste

1 1/2 cups shredded reduced-fat Swiss cheese, divided

In a mixing bowl beat eggs and egg whites with milk, mustard, salt, and pepper; set aside. Place half the bread slices in a 13×9×2-inch baking dish coated with nonstick cooking spray. In a skillet coated with nonstick cooking spray, sauté the mushrooms, garlic, and onion until tender. Add the spinach and flour, stirring to mix well. Season with salt and pepper to taste. Spread mixture over bread. Sprinkle with 1 cup cheese. Top with remaining bread. Sprinkle with remaining 1/2 cup cheese. Pour egg mixture over casserole and refrigerate 2 hours or overnight. Bake at 350 degrees for 40 to 50 minutes or until puffed and golden.

Nutritional information per serving

Calories 240, Protein (g) 16, Carbohydrate (g) 28, Fat (g) 7, Cal. from Fat (%) 26, Saturated Fat (g) 3, Dietary Fiber (g) 3, Cholesterol (mg) 101, Sodium (mg) 482, Diabetic Exchanges: 1 very lean meat, 1.5 starch, 1 vegetable, 1 fat

DOC'S NOTES:

This is a great dish to try several days before your next cycle of treatment. Good source of vitamins and minerals.

Egg Soufflé 🥕

Leave out the pepper and onions for a plain version of a cheesy egg dish.

MAKES 12 SERVINGS

7 slices whole wheat bread, crusts removed
1 red bell pepper, cored and chopped
1 bunch green onions (scallions), chopped
6 ounces reduced fat sharp Cheddar
 cheese, shredded
6 ounces reduced fat Monterey Jack cheese,
 shredded
5 large eggs
4 large egg whites
3 cups skim milk
2 tablespoons margarine, melted
1 teaspoon dry mustard
1 teaspoon Worcestershire sauce, optional
Salt and pepper to taste

Preheat oven to 350 degrees. Line bottom of a 3-quart or 13×9×2-inch baking dish with slices of bread. Cover with chopped red peppers and green onions. Sprinkle with shredded cheeses. In bowl, mix remaining ingredients and pour mixture over cheeses. Refrigerate for 6 hours or overnight. Bake for 45 minutes to 1 hour.

Nutritional information per serving

Calories 197, Protein (g) 16, Carbohydrate (g) 11, Fat (g) 10, Cal. from Fat (%) 45, Saturated Fat (g) 4, Dietary Fiber (g) 1, Cholesterol (mg) 105, Sodium (mg) 358, Diabetic Exchanges: 2 lean meat, 0.5 starch, 1 fat

DOC'S NOTES:

This is a great breakfast dish. You might cut this recipe in half. Breakfast foods seem to be the best tolerated of all foods while you are having chemotherapy.

Egg Noodle Casserole 🥕

The simple combination of noodles, eggs, and a white sauce translate into a great breakfast dish that can be made ahead.

MAKES 6 SERVINGS

1 (8-ounce) package wide noodles
1/4 cup all-purpose flour
2 cups skim milk
1 teaspoon Worcestershire sauce
Salt and pepper to taste
1/2 teaspoon garlic powder
6 hard-boiled large eggs, whites only, chopped
2/3 cup shredded reduced-fat Cheddar cheese

Preheat oven to 350 degrees. Cook the noodles according to package directions, omitting any salt and oil. Drain; set aside. In a small saucepan, mix together the flour and milk. Cook over a medium heat, stirring, until thickened. Add the Worcestershire sauce, salt and pepper, and garlic powder. Arrange half of the egg whites in the bottom of a 2-quart casserole dish coated with nonstick cooking spray. Cover the egg whites with half of the noodles, then add half the cheese, then half the white sauce. Repeat layers. Bake for 30 minutes.

Nutritional information per serving
*Calories 245, Protein (g) 16, Carbohydrate (g) 36,
Fat (g) 4, Cal. from Fat (%) 15, Saturated Fat (g) 2,
Dietary Fiber (g) 1, Cholesterol (mg) 44, Sodium (mg) 194,
Diabetic Exchanges: 1 lean meat, 2 starch, 0.5 skim milk*

DOC'S NOTES:

Use this dish for breakfast, lunch, or dinner. Remember, if it appeals to you at the time, it is OK to eat it whenever. The eggs provide a great source of protein, vitamins, and minerals while the cheese adds protein and calcium.

Crabmeat Egg Casserole

Crabmeat lovers will enjoy this delicious brunch dish. White or claw crabmeat can be used. Adjust the chopped veggies to what you can tolerate.

MAKES 10 SERVINGS

6 slices whole wheat bread
1/2 cup water
1 tablespoon margarine, melted
1 onion, chopped
1/2 cup chopped green bell pepper
1/2 cup chopped celery
2 cloves garlic, minced
8 ounces reduced fat sharp Cheddar
    cheese, shredded
1 pound lump crabmeat, picked for bones
1 large egg
2 large egg whites
1/2 cup nonfat plain yogurt
Salt and pepper to taste

Preheat oven to 350 degrees. Place bread in a bowl with 1/2 cup water. Let stand 15 minutes. In a skillet coated with nonstick cooking spray, melt margarine and sauté onion, green pepper, celery, and garlic until tender. Add shredded cheese to bread and water mixture, stirring together. Carefully stir in sautéed vegetables, and crabmeat. In a mixing bowl, beat egg, egg whites, yogurt, and salt and pepper. Combine with crabmeat mixture, mixing well. Transfer into a 2-quart baking dish and bake for 30 to 40 minutes.

Nutritional information per serving

Calories 205, Protein (g) 21, Carbohydrate (g) 14, Fat (g) 7, Cal. from Fat (%) 31, Saturated Fat (g) 3, Dietary Fiber (g) 3, Cholesterol (mg) 68, Sodium (mg) 454, Diabetic Exchanges: 2.5 lean meat, 0.5 starch, 1 vegetable

DOC'S NOTES:

This is a meal in one. Add a fruit salad and you are set for the day!

Strawberry Soup

*Strawberries offer a high antioxidant profile
and vitamin C.*

MAKES FIVE (1-CUP) SERVINGS

1 quart strawberries, hulled
Juice of 1 orange
3 tablespoons confectioners' sugar
1 (12-ounce) can peach nectar
1½ cups nonfat plain yogurt

In a food processor, combine strawberries
and orange juice; blend until smooth.
Add the sugar. Gradually add the peach
nectar, blending well. Add yogurt, blending
until mixed. Refrigerate.

Nutritional information per serving

*Calories 139, Protein (g) 5, Carbohydrate (g) 30,
Fat (g) 1, Cal. from Fat (%) 4, Saturated Fat (g) 0,
Dietary Fiber (g) 3, Cholesterol (mg) 1, Sodium (mg) 63,
Diabetic Exchanges: 1.5 fruit, 0.5 skim milk*

Peach Soup

Canned peaches may be used.

MAKES 10 SERVINGS

1½ pounds peaches, peeled, pitted and sliced
2 cups nonfat plain yogurt
1 cup orange juice
1 cup pineapple juice
1 tablespoon lemon juice
2 tablespoons sugar
¼ cup sherry, optional

Purée peaches in a food processor until
smooth. Add all remaining ingredients and
blend well. Refrigerate to serve chilled.

Nutritional information per serving

*Calories 89, Protein (g) 3, Carbohydrate (g) 18,
Fat (g) 0, Cal. from Fat (%) 0, Saturated Fat (g) 0,
Dietary Fiber (g) 1, Cholesterol (mg) 0, Sodium (mg) 39,
Diabetic Exchanges: 1 fruit, 0.5 skim milk*

DOC'S NOTES:

A light lunch; goes well 2 to 3 days post
chemotherapy.

DOC'S NOTES:

Source of Vitamin C, calcium, protein,
riboflavin, phosphorus, and B12.

Asparagus and Potato Soup 🥕 ❄️

By combining the ever popular potato soup with asparagus, you have a glorious creation. Serve hot or cold.

MAKES EIGHT (1-CUP) SERVINGS

4 cups diced peeled red potatoes (about 3)
1 cup chopped onion
4 (14½-ounce) cans cut asparagus, drained, reserving liquid
1 teaspoon minced garlic
1 (12-ounce) can evaporated skimmed milk
Salt and pepper to taste

In a large pot, combine potatoes and onion in salted water and bring to a boil. Reduce heat and cook about 15 minutes or until tender, drain. Drain cans of asparagus, reserving the juice from two of the cans. Combine potatoes, onion, asparagus, and garlic in large bowl. Using a food processor, process the asparagus/potato mixture in batches until entire mixture is puréed. Add the milk, reserved asparagus juice if needed to thin, and salt and pepper. Refrigerate.

Nutritional information per serving
*Calories 136, Protein (g) 9, Carbohydrate (g) 26,
Fat (g) 1, Cal. from Fat (%) 4, Saturated Fat (g) 0,
Dietary Fiber (g) 4, Cholesterol (mg) 2, Sodium (mg) 644,
Diabetic Exchanges: 1 starch, 0.5 skim milk, 1 vegetable*

DOC'S NOTES:

Rich in Vitamin C.

Chicken Soup ❄

Chicken soup is healing and also freezes well. To reduce the sodium, leave out some or all of the bouillon cubes.

MAKES EIGHT TO TEN (1-CUP) SERVINGS

4 quarts water
3 pounds skinless, boneless chicken breasts,
  cut into pieces
1 large onion, cut into wedges
6 sprigs of parsley
3 bay leaves
2 cloves garlic, halved
1 (16-ounce) package baby carrots
1 cup chopped celery
1 turnip, cut into chunks
Salt and pepper to taste
4 chicken bouillon cubes
Cooked rice or noodles, optional

Place all ingredients except rice or noodles in a large pot. Bring to a boil. Reduce the heat, cover, and simmer 45 minutes, or until the chicken is tender. If desired, remove the chicken, carrots, celery, and turnip from the broth and strain the soup. Add the rice or noodles, if desired, and heat through.

Nutritional information per serving

Calories 188, Protein (g) 33, Carbohydrate (g) 8, Fat (g) 2, Cal. from Fat (%) 12, Saturated Fat (g) 1, Dietary Fiber (g) 2, Cholesterol (mg) 79, Sodium (mg) 570, Diabetic Exchanges: 4 very lean meat, 1.5 vegetable0

DOC'S NOTES:

This makes a great meal 3 to 4 days following chemotherapy.

Chicken, Barley, and Bow-Tie Soup ❄

This hearty version of a favorite remedy with barley and pasta quickly became a favorite in my house.

MAKES 10 TO 12 SERVINGS

2½ pounds skinless, boneless chicken breasts,
  cut into 1-inch pieces
1 cup chopped celery
1½ cups chopped onion
2 cups thinly sliced carrots
1 bay leaf
12 cups water
½ cup pearl barley
Salt and pepper to taste
½ teaspoon dried basil leaves
3 chicken bouillon cubes
1 (16-ounce) package bow-tie pasta

Place the chicken, celery, onion, carrots, bay leaf, and 12 cups water in a large pot. Bring to a boil and add the barley. Reduce the heat, cover, and cook until the chicken and barley are done, about 30 minutes. Season with salt and pepper, and add the basil and bouillon cubes. Meanwhile, cook the pasta according to package directions, omitting oil and salt. Drain and set aside. Remove the bay leaf and add the pasta.

Nutritional information per serving
*Calories 296, Protein (g) 28, Carbohydrate (g) 39,
Fat (g) 2, Cal. from Fat (%) 7, Saturated Fat (g) 1,
Dietary Fiber (g) 3, Cholesterol (mg) 55, Sodium (mg) 360,
Diabetic Exchanges: 2.5 very lean meat, 2.5 starch,
1 vegetable*

DOC'S NOTES:

This goes great any time post-treatment. Barley is a whole grain and a high fiber substitute for rice or pasta.

Fruity Couscous Salad 🥕

Couscous is made from semolina and is found in your local grocery store. Couscous is easily prepared to create this wonderful salad.

MAKES 8 CUPS, 10 TO 12 SERVINGS

2 cups canned fat-free chicken broth

2 cups couscous

1/2 cup dried tart cherries or dried cranberries

2/3 cup coarsely chopped carrots

1 cup chopped unpeeled cucumber

1 bunch green onions (scallions), chopped

1/4 cup pine nuts or slivered almonds,
   toasted, optional

3 tablespoons balsamic vinegar

1 tablespoon olive oil

1 tablespoon Dijon mustard

Salt and pepper to taste

Bring broth to a boil in a medium saucepan; stir in couscous. Remove from heat; let stand, covered, 5 minutes. Fluff with a fork. Uncover; cool 10 minutes. Combine cooked couscous, dried fruit, carrots, cucumber, green onions, and pine nuts in a large bowl; mix well. Combine vinegar, olive oil, and mustard in a small bowl; mix well. Pour dressing mixture over couscous mixture; stir to coat all ingredients. Season with salt and pepper, if desired. Serve chilled or at room temperature.

Nutritional information per serving

Calories 144, Protein (g) 5, Carbohydrate (g) 29, Fat (g) 1, Cal. from Fat (%) 8, Saturated Fat (g) 0, Dietary Fiber (g) 2, Cholesterol (mg) 0, Sodium (mg) 141, Diabetic Exchanges: 1.5 starch, 0.5 fruit

DOC'S NOTES:

Carrots provide potassium and beta carotene. Carrots may lower blood cholesterol. The dried fruit also adds fiber and potassium.

Waldorf Pasta Salad

This light colorful salad is like eating a fruit salad with pasta. Top with grilled chicken for a hearty salad.

MAKES 6 SERVINGS

8 ounces bow tie pasta
1 cup nonfat plain yogurt
¼ cup frozen orange juice concentrate
1 (11-ounce) can mandarin orange slices, drained
1 cup seedless red grapes, halved
1 green apple, cored and chopped
1 cup chopped celery

Prepare the pasta according to package directions; set aside. In a small bowl, blend the yogurt with the orange juice. In a large bowl, combine the pasta, mandarin orange slices, grapes, apple, and celery. Stir in the yogurt mixture; toss well. Cover and refrigerate until chilled.

Nutritional information per serving

Calories 235, Protein (g) 8, Carbohydrate (g) 50,
Fat (g) 1, Cal. from Fat (%) 3, Saturated Fat (g) 0,
Dietary Fiber (g) 3, Cholesterol (mg) 1, Sodium (mg) 53,
Diabetic Exchanges: 2 starch, 1 fruit, 0.5 skim milk

DOC'S NOTES:

This is a full meal in one dish. The fruit are great sources of fiber. Red grapes are a source of resveratrol which is a phytochemical or cancer protective substance.

Tuna Salad

Canned tuna turned into a delightful dish.

MAKES 8 SERVINGS

2 (6-ounce) cans white tuna, packed in
   water, drained
1 (11-ounce) can mandarin oranges, drained
1/4 pound fresh mushrooms, sliced
1 (14-ounce) can artichoke hearts, drained and
   cut in half
1 (8-ounce) can sliced water chestnuts, drained

Carefully combine all ingredients in large
bowl. Toss with Dressing (recipe follows).
Serve immediately.

DRESSING

1/4 cup fat-free or light mayonnaise
1/4 cup nonfat plain yogurt
1 tablespoon lemon juice
1 teaspoon sugar
1 bunch green onions (scallions), chopped

Combine all ingredients together and fold
into tuna mixture.

Nutritional information per serving

Calories 108, Protein (g) 12, Carbohydrate (g) 11,
Fat (g) 2, Cal. from Fat (%) 14, Saturated Fat (g) 0,
Dietary Fiber (g) 3, Cholesterol (mg) 19, Sodium (mg) 324,
Diabetic Exchanges: 1.5 very lean meat, 2 vegetable

DOC'S NOTES:

Great salad on those hot summer days.
Good source of fiber, Vitamin C, B,
copper, and other minerals.

Perfect Pasta

Takes angel hair to a new level.

MAKES 6 TO 8 SERVINGS

1 (12-ounce) package angel hair pasta
3 tablespoons olive oil
2 cloves garlic, minced
1 tablespoon finely chopped parsley

Cook pasta according to directions on package, omitting salt and oil. Drain and set aside. In a small pan, combine all remaining ingredients and sauté for a few minutes. Pour over cooked pasta and toss. Serve immediately.

Nutritional information per serving

Calories 204, Protein (g) 6, Carbohydrate (g) 32,
Fat (g) 6, Cal. from Fat (%) 26, Saturated Fat (g) 1,
Dietary Fiber (g) 1, Cholesterol (mg) 0, Sodium (mg) 3,
Diabetic Exchanges: 1 starch, 1 fat

DOC'S NOTES:

Good anytime post-treatment.

Potato Pizza

Instead of mashed or baked potatoes, try this version. Adjust the recipe for your family by adding different cheeses or leaving off the onions. . .serve with a dollop of plain yogurt.

MAKES 6 TO 8 SERVINGS

4 baking potatoes, peeled and cut into 1/4-inch
   thick round slices
1 tablespoon minced garlic
2 tablespoons olive oil
Salt and pepper to taste
1/2 cup chopped green onions (scallions)
1/2 cup shredded reduced-fat Cheddar cheese

Preheat oven to 350 degrees. In a large bowl, mix together the potato slices, garlic, olive oil, and salt and pepper. Coat a 12-inch pizza pan with nonstick cooking spray and arrange the potato slices to cover the pizza pan, overlapping the slices. Bake for 35 to 40 minutes or until the potato slices are tender. Remove from the oven and sprinkle with the green onions and cheese. Return to the oven and continue baking 5 minutes longer or until the cheese is melted.

Nutritional information per serving

Calories 104, Protein (g) 4, Carbohydrate (g) 14, Fat (g) 5, Cal. from Fat (%) 37, Saturated Fat (g) 1, Dietary Fiber (g) 2, Cholesterol (mg) 4, Sodium (mg) 46, Diabetic Exchanges: 1 starch, 1 fat

Cheesy Macaroni

A comfort food that we are never too old to enjoy. The cheeses are high in calcium and protein. Add more milk if needed to thin.

MAKES 8 SERVINGS

1 (16-ounce) package elbow macaroni

2 tablespoons cornstarch

2 cups skim milk

1 (8-ounce) package reduced-fat sharp Cheddar cheese, cut into chunks

1 (16-ounce) container reduced fat cottage cheese

Salt and pepper to taste

Cook pasta according to package directions, drain. In a large pot, mix together cornstarch and milk over medium heat, stirring until thickened. Add Cheddar cheese, stirring until melted. Add pasta, tossing until well combined and heated. In a food processor, blend cottage cheese until smooth. Add to pasta mixture. Season with salt and pepper.

Nutritional information per serving

Calories 360, Protein (g) 24, Carbohydrate (g) 49, Fat (g) 7, Cal. from Fat (%) 17, Saturated Fat (g) 4, Dietary Fiber (g) 1, Cholesterol (mg) 24, Sodium (mg) 405, Diabetic Exchanges: 2 lean meat, 3 starch, 0.5 skim milk

DOC'S NOTES:

A higher calorie and good source of protein and calcium recipe. This makes a great light main dish.

Orzo Asparagus Toss

Asparagus adds spunk to this Italian pasta dish. Orzo is a rice shaped pasta. Substitute any pasta for this dish.

MAKES 6 SERVINGS

1 (16-ounce) package orzo

2 tablespoons olive oil

2 cups asparagus spears, cut in 2-inch pieces

1 red bell pepper, cored and cut in strips

1 cup thinly sliced onion

1 tablespoon finely minced garlic

1 cup tomato chunks

1/3 cup grated Romano cheese, optional

Cook orzo according to directions on package. Drain and set aside. Meanwhile, in a large skillet, heat olive oil and sauté the asparagus, red pepper, onion, garlic, and tomato until all are tender. Add cooked orzo and toss together. If desired, add the Romano cheese.

Nutritional information per serving

Calories 354, Protein (g) 12, Carbohydrate (g) 64, Fat (g) 6, Cal. from Fat (%) 15, Saturated Fat (g) 1, Dietary Fiber (g) 4, Cholesterol (mg) 0, Sodium (mg) 10, Diabetic Exchanges: 4 starch, 1 vegetable, 0.5 fat

DOC'S NOTES:

This is another healthful, easy to fix meal and adjust pepper, onion, and tomato to how you feel. Serve with grilled chicken breast and whole wheat toast for a complete meal.

Simply Delicious Chicken ❄

When I was testing recipes my family made me promise to repeat this dish often. The simplicity of the dish is very appealing.

MAKES 8 SERVINGS

2 pounds boneless skinless chicken breasts
1/3 cup all-purpose flour
Salt and pepper to taste
2 tablespoons olive oil
1 cup canned fat-free chicken broth
1 tablespoon cornstarch
Juice of 1/2 lemon
2 tablespoons chopped parsley

Dust the chicken breasts with flour and salt and pepper. In large skillet, sauté the chicken in olive oil until brown and almost done. Mix together the chicken broth and cornstarch; add to the skillet. Stir in the lemon juice. Sprinkle with parsley before serving.

Nutritional information per serving
Calories 180, Protein (g) 27, Carbohydrate (g) 5, Fat (g) 5, Cal. from Fat (%) 25, Saturated Fat (g) 1, Dietary Fiber (g) 0, Cholesterol (mg) 66, Sodium (mg) 152, Diabetic Exchanges: 3 very lean meat, 0.5 starch

DOC'S NOTES:

Nutritious yet simple and elegant and low fat. Anyone in the house can prepare this main course.

Chicken Diane with Wild Rice ❄

This light chicken entrée has the taste and flair of a gourmet dish without all the complication. Mushrooms are nutritious; they contain some protein, vitamins, and minerals. Try using the different varieties.

MAKES 4 TO 6 SERVINGS

3/4 pound mushrooms, sliced

1 cup chopped onion

1½ pounds skinless, boneless chicken breasts

Salt and pepper to taste

1/4 cup chopped green onion (scallion) stems (green part only)

2 tablespoons chopped parsley

1 cup canned fat-free chicken broth

3 tablespoons sherry, optional

1½ tablespoons Dijon mustard

1 (6-ounce) box long-grain and wild rice

1 (14-ounce) can artichoke heart quarters, drained

Coat a large skillet with nonstick cooking spray and sauté the mushrooms and onion over medium heat until tender, about 5 minutes. Remove from the skillet; set aside. Sprinkle the chicken breasts with salt and pepper. In the same skillet coated with nonstick cooking spray, cook the chicken until lightly browned on both sides, about 5 to 7 minutes.

Spoon the reserved mushroom mixture over the chicken in the pan. Combine the green onions, parsley, chicken broth, sherry, and Dijon mustard in a small bowl and pour over the chicken. Cover, reduce the heat, and simmer 20 minutes or until the chicken is tender. Meanwhile, prepare the rice according to the package directions. Toss the cooked rice with the artichoke hearts. Serve the chicken and sauce on top of the rice.

Nutritional information per serving

Calories 274, Protein (g) 32, Carbohydrate (g) 30, Fat (g) 2, Cal. from Fat (%) 6, Saturated Fat (g) 0, Dietary Fiber (g) 2, Cholesterol (mg) 66, Sodium (mg) 810, Diabetic Exchanges: 3 very lean meat, 1.5 starch, 1.5 vegetable

DOC'S NOTES:

A little sherry will not hurt you. Enjoy!

Italian Chicken

This is way too easy to be so good! The Italian herbs give that finishing touch.

MAKES 4 SERVINGS

1 (6-ounce) box long grain and wild rice mix
3/4 cup water
1 (14 1/2-ounce) can diced tomatoes
1/2 cup shredded part-skim mozzarella cheese
2 teaspoons dried basil leaves, divided
2 teaspoons dried oregano leaves, divided
1 teaspoon minced garlic
1 1/2 pounds skinless, boneless chicken breasts, cut into strips
1/4 cup grated Parmesan cheese

Preheat oven to 375 degrees. In a 2- to 3-quart oblong baking dish coated with nonstick cooking spray, combine the water, rice, seasoning packet, tomatoes, mozzarella, 1 teaspoon basil, 1 teaspoon oregano, and garlic, stirring well. Top the rice mixture with the chicken strips and sprinkle with the remaining basil and oregano and the Parmesan cheese. Bake, covered, for 45 minutes. Uncover and continue baking 15 minutes longer, or until the chicken is tender and the rice is cooked.

Nutritional information per serving

Calories 430, Protein (g) 50, Carbohydrate (g) 40, Fat (g) 7, Cal. from Fat (%) 14, Saturated Fat (g) 3.2, Dietary Fiber (g) 3, Cholesterol (mg) 112, Sodium (mg) 1055, Diabetic Exchanges: 5 very lean meat, 2.5 starch, 1 vegetable

DOC'S NOTES:

This is a great one-dish meal to enjoy during the week prior to your next treatment.

Quick Chicken and Dumplings ❄

The flour tortillas are a great trick to use for no-trouble dumplings and will enhance the chicken soup.

MAKES 8 TO 10 SERVINGS

5¼ cups canned fat-free chicken broth
5¼ cups water
1½ pounds boneless skinless chicken breasts, cut into pieces
1 cup sliced carrots
Salt and pepper to taste
10 (6-inch) flour or whole wheat tortillas

Pour the chicken broth and water into a large pot. Add the chicken pieces, carrots, and salt and pepper to taste. Bring the mixture to a boil. Reduce the heat to medium and continue to cook for 25 minutes or until the chicken is done and the carrots are tender. Cut the tortillas into small wedges. Add the cut up tortillas to the pot and stir. Continue to cook until the tortillas are tender, about 5 minutes. If you need more liquid in pot, add more broth or water.

Nutritional information per serving
*Calories 178, Protein (g) 20, Carbohydrate (g) 15,
Fat (g) 4, Cal. from Fat (%) 20, Saturated Fat (g) 0,
Dietary Fiber (g) 0, Cholesterol (mg) 40, Sodium (mg) 598,
Diabetic Exchanges: 2 very lean meat, 1 starch*

DOC'S NOTES:

Light and hearty — enjoy at any time during your chemotherapy cycle.

Baked Fish

Another quick topping that is outstanding on any fish!

MAKES 4 SERVINGS

1 pound fish fillets
2 tablespoons light mayonnaise or
   mayonnaise of choice
1 teaspoon lemon juice
1/2 teaspoon prepared mustard
1/2 teaspoon sugar
1/4 teaspoon Worcestershire sauce
1/4 teaspoon onion powder
1/4 teaspoon garlic powder
1/8 teaspoon cayenne pepper, optional
Paprika

Rinse fish and pat dry. In a small dish combine remaining ingredients except paprika, mixing well. Lay fish in an oblong baking dish coated with nonstick cooking spray. Spread mayonnaise mixture over fillets. Marinate 30 minutes. Preheat oven to 500 degrees. Sprinkle with paprika. Bake for 10 to 15 minutes or until fish flakes easily with fork.

Nutritional information per serving

Calories 122, Protein (g) 20, Carbohydrate (g) 2,
Fat (g) 3, Cal. from Fat (%) 25, Saturated Fat (g) 1,
Dietary Fiber (g) 0, Cholesterol (mg) 51, Sodium (mg) 133,
Diabetic Exchanges: 3 very lean meat

DOC'S NOTES:

This is light and easily digested. Great replacement for red meat. Some drugs make you lose your taste for red meat.

Broiled Shrimp

When you want a delicious recipe with no clean up, here it is. The pan is lined with foil and no other dishes are used. No effort, yet great taste.

MAKES 8 SERVINGS

2 pounds peeled large shrimp
1 tablespoon minced garlic
1/3 cup balsamic vinegar
1/4 cup white wine, optional
1/2 cup Italian bread crumbs
1/4 cup grated Parmesan cheese
2 tablespoons olive oil

Preheat the broiler. Lay shrimp on a foil-lined pan. Sprinkle with the garlic, vinegar, and white wine. Sprinkle bread crumbs and Parmesan cheese on top. Drizzle with the olive oil. Let sit for 15 minutes. Place under broiler for about 10 to 15 minutes or until shrimp are done. Watch carefully while cooking.

Nutritional information per serving

Calories 203, Protein (g) 25, Carbohydrate (g) 9, Fat (g) 7, Cal. from Fat (%) 31, Saturated Fat (g) 1, Dietary Fiber (g) 0, Cholesterol (mg) 175, Sodium (mg) 336, Diabetic Exchanges: 3 very lean meat, 0.5 starch, 1 fat

DOC'S NOTES:

Great dish to have the week before the next cycle of chemotherapy is scheduled. Serve with a simple green salad, French bread, and a glass of white wine. Shrimp are low in calories and are an excellent source of protein, iron, and trace minerals zinc and copper.

Yam Biscuits

You can quickly whip up these biscuits with ingredients found in your pantry. By including yams, you're including nutrition. Make larger biscuits to use for sandwiches.

MAKES 2 DOZEN

1 (15-ounce) can sweet potatoes (yams), drained and mashed
4 cups all-purpose baking mix
1/2 teaspoon ground cinnamon
3/4 cup skim milk
3 tablespoons margarine, softened

Preheat oven to 450 degrees. In a mixing bowl, mix the mashed yams with the baking mix and cinnamon. Add the milk and margarine to the mixture, stirring until blended. Roll on a floured surface to 1-inch thickness. Cut with a 2-inch cutter or a glass and place on a baking sheet. Bake for 10 to 12 minutes or until golden brown.

Nutritional information per serving

Calories 110, Protein (g) 2, Carbohydrate (g) 16, Fat (g) 5, Cal. from Fat (%) 36, Saturated Fat (g) 1, Dietary Fiber (g) 1, Cholesterol (mg) 0, Sodium (mg) 282, Diabetic Exchanges: 1 starch, 1 fat

DOC'S NOTES:

Sweet potatoes are rich in beta carotene, and Vitamins C and B.

Chess Pie 🥕 ❄️

Whip up this quick yummy pie when you have a sweet tooth, but want something not too rich. Add lemon extract for a lemon flavor.

MAKES 6 TO 8 SERVINGS

2 tablespoons margarine, melted
1 cup sugar
3 tablespoons all-purpose flour
1 (5-ounce) can evaporated skimmed milk
2 large eggs, beaten
1 teaspoon butter extract
1 (9-inch) pie shell, unbaked

Preheat oven to 350 degrees. Combine the margarine, sugar, flour, evaporated milk, eggs, and butter extract in a bowl, beating well. Pour into the pie shell. Bake for 30 minutes or until firm. Cool before serving.

Nutritional information per serving
Calories 249, Protein (g) 4, Carbohydrate (g) 39, Fat (g) 9, Cal. from Fat (%) 31, Saturated Fat (g) 3, Dietary Fiber (g) 0, Cholesterol (mg) 57, Sodium (mg) 132, Diabetic Exchanges: 1 starch, 1.5 other carb., 1.5 fat

DOC'S NOTES:

A slice or two daily for lunch or dinner will help keep your weight up.

Banana Pudding Trifle 🥕

For a quicker version, use instant vanilla pudding or sugar-free instant pudding. However, I love a homemade custard pudding so I included the option. English toffee may be omitted, if desired, but it sure makes this trifle good.

MAKES 16 SERVINGS

2/3 cup sugar

3/4 cup all-purpose flour

3 1/2 cups skim milk

2 large egg yolks, slightly beaten

1 tablespoon vanilla extract

1 (11-ounce) box reduced-fat vanilla wafers, divided

6 bananas, divided

2 (1.4-ounce) English toffee candy bars, crushed, divided

1 (8-ounce) container fat-free frozen whipped topping, thawed

In a large saucepan, combine the sugar and flour. Gradually stir in the milk and bring the mixture to a boil over a medium-high heat, stirring constantly. Place the egg yolks in a small bowl and gradually pour some of the hot custard into the egg yolks, mixing well with a fork. Gradually pour the hot custard mixture back into the saucepan with the remaining custard, cooking over a low heat for several minutes. Do not boil. Remove from the heat and add the vanilla. Transfer the custard to a bowl and allow to cool (can refrigerate to speed up the cooling). In a trifle bowl or large glass bowl, place one-third of the vanilla wafers. Slice 2 of the bananas and place on top the wafers. Spread one-half of the custard on top and sprinkle with one-half of the crushed candy bars. Repeat the layers again using all of the remaining custard and crushed candy bars. Place the final one-third of the vanilla wafers on top. Slice 2 bananas on top of wafers and cover with the whipped topping. Refrigerate at least 1 hour before serving.

Nutritional information per serving

Calories 255, Protein (g) 4, Carbohydrate (g) 50, Fat (g) 4, Cal. from Fat (%) 14, Saturated Fat (g) 1, Dietary Fiber (g) 1, Cholesterol (mg) 30, Sodium (mg) 121, Diabetic Exchanges: 1.5 starch, 1 fruit, 1 other carb., 0.5 fat

DOC'S NOTES:

This is an excellent source of potassium.

Lemon Angel Food Cake 🥕

Serve this cake with assorted fresh berries or a fruit sauce. As a time saver, you can use a commercially prepared angel food cake and just omit lemon extract.

MAKES 12 SERVINGS

1 (16-ounce) box angel food cake mix
1 teaspoon lemon extract
1 (6-serving) package vanilla pudding mix
1 (8-ounce) container nonfat lemon yogurt
1 (8-ounce) container fat free frozen whipped
  topping, thawed

Prepare cake according to package directions and adding lemon extract. Bake as directed in an angel food cake pan. Cool upside down over a narrow-neck bottle. In a bowl, blend dry pudding mix with lemon yogurt using a wire whisk. Fold in whipped topping. Remove cake from pan. Slice cake horizontally into 3 layers. Place bottom layer on a serving plate and top with one-third of lemon yogurt mixture. Repeat layers twice. Refrigerate.

Nutritional information per serving

Calories 227, Protein (g) 4, Carbohydrate (g) 51, Fat (g) 0, Cal. from Fat (%) 0, Saturated Fat (g) 0, Dietary Fiber (g) 0, Cholesterol (mg) 0, Sodium (mg) 329, Diabetic Exchanges: 1.5 starch, 2 other carb.

DOC'S NOTES:

Tasty yet very healthful and low in fat.

Mock Chocolate Eclair 🥕

Requests for graham crackers and pudding put this recipe high on your list.

MAKES 15 TO 20 SERVINGS

2 wrapped packages graham crackers
   (from 16-ounce box)
2 (4-serving) packages vanilla instant pudding
   and pie filling
3 cups skim milk
1/2 (8-ounce) container frozen fat-free
   whipped topping

Layer bottom of a 13×9×2-inch baking dish with one-third of graham crackers. In a mixing bowl, beat pudding mix with milk until thickened; let stand for several minutes. Fold in whipped topping. Spread half of pudding mixture over graham crackers. Repeat layers, ending with graham crackers on top (three layers graham crackers). Spread with Chocolate Topping (recipe follows).

CHOCOLATE TOPPING

1/4 cup cocoa
1/3 cup sugar
1/4 cup skim milk
1 tablespoon vanilla extract
1 tablespoon margarine

Combine cocoa, sugar, and milk in a saucepan. Bring to a boil for 1 minute. Remove from heat and add vanilla and margarine. Cool slightly and pour over graham crackers. Refrigerate until ready to serve (can be made night before).

Nutritional information per serving
Calories 144, Protein (g) 3, Carbohydrate (g) 28, Fat (g) 2, Cal. from Fat (%) 14, Saturated Fat (g) 0, Dietary Fiber (g) 1, Cholesterol (mg) 1, Sodium (mg) 252, Diabetic Exchanges: 2 starch

DOC'S NOTES:

Eat this seven days a week. Easy on the tummy anytime.

Neutropenia
(LOW WHITE BLOOD CELL COUNT)

◆ What is neutropenia?

◆ Do I have to go into isolation?

◆ How long does neutropenia last?

◆ Is it okay to eat raw fruits and vegetables once neutropenia has subsided?

Neutropenia, or low white blood cell count, is a common complication following a large number of treatments. Most chemotherapeutic drugs will lower your blood counts to some degree. This is because chemotherapy will destroy good cells such as white blood cells, red blood cells and platelets that are produced in the bone marrow. Our goal with chemotherapy is to destroy cancer cells and allow good cells to regenerate and flourish. Unfortunately, we destroy both good and bad cells after each treatment of chemotherapy. The nausea and vomiting is partially secondary to the destruction of cells lining the gastrointestinal tract. Hair loss is secondary to the destruction of hair follicles.

Neutropenia usually lasts four to seven days. This can vary from person to person and treatment to treatment. Normally, we recommend avoiding crowds and anyone that is ill until your blood counts are normal. Raw fruits, vegetables, meat, and seafood are harbingers of bacteria which, if ingested during the times your white blood cells are low, can lead to a systemic infection and should also be avoided. You can become neutropenic following successive treatments. The neutropenia will only last four to seven days in most cases; however, it can be longer with certain leukemia treatments. Once your counts have recovered you can resume your normal activities and diet.

Again during the period of neutropenia, avoid raw fruits, raw vegetables, raw meat and raw seafood. I hope the recipes that follow will give you directions on what to eat during the time your white blood cell count is down and you are more susceptible to infections.

Shopping List for Neutropenia
- Butter or margarine
- Bread
- Cheese
- Canned broth
- Dried seasonings and spices
- Eggs
- Fruit, canned
- Grits
- Milk, skim
- Oatmeal
- Pasta
- Potatoes
- Skinless boneless chicken breasts
- Vegetables, canned, frozen, fresh must be cooked
- Yogurt
- Whipped topping, frozen

Points to Remember
- NO RAW FOOD
- Cooked fruit or veggies
- No fresh, frozen, or dried fruit
- No honey – use molasses
- Avoid uncooked herbs and spices
- Processed cheese is acceptable
- Canned or cooked fruits are acceptable
- All cooked or baked goods, jello, syrup, ice cream and sherbet made from pasteurized products are acceptable
- Yogurt
- Cooked hot soups
- All breads, rolls, crackers in wrappers

Menus

Foods to eat when neutropenia is occurring.

Breakfast

224   Oatmeal Pancakes

22   Cinnamon Rolls

26   Apple Lasagna
56   Quick Cheese Grits

25   Baked French Toast

Lunch

57   Pumpkin Soup *or*
59   Two-Potato Bisque

65   Chicken Pot Pie
68   Hot Fruit Compote

Dinner

Chicken Piccata   66
Linguine Florentine   62
Mocha Cappuccino Pudding Pie   70

Baked Topped Fish   247
Cheesy Macaroni   40
Chess Pie   49

Very Good Veal   67
Carrot Soufflé   140

Egg Noodle Casserole   29
Baked Peach Delight   71

Snacks

Cheese Quesadillas   193

Artichoke Squares   187

Hot Cocoa Drink Supplement   74
or Awesome Milkshake   146

Mini Cheese Pizzas   189

Quick Cheese Grits

NEUTROPENIA

MAKES 12 SERVINGS

Sometimes grits just hit the spot. If not serving immediately, reheat, and add milk to make creamy if needed.

4 cups water
1 cup skim milk
1/2 teaspoon salt
1 1/2 cups quick grits
3 tablespoons margarine
3 cups shredded reduced-fat Cheddar cheese
1 tablespoon Worcestershire sauce
1/4 teaspoon garlic powder

In a saucepan, bring the water, milk, and salt to a boil. Add grits, reduce heat, and cook about 5 minutes, stirring occasionally. Add margarine, cheese, Worcestershire sauce, and garlic powder. Stir until margarine and cheese melts.

Nutritional information per serving

Calories 186, Protein (g) 11, Carbohydrate (g) 17, Fat (g) 8, Cal. from Fat (%) 40, Saturated Fat (g) 4, Dietary Fiber (g) 0, Cholesterol (mg) 15, Sodium (mg) 335, Diabetic Exchanges: 1 lean meat, 1 starch, 1 fat

DOC'S NOTES:

For weight gain, don't used reduced-fat products.

Pumpkin Soup ▧ ❄

Here's a quick soup that is especially perfect to serve in the fall.

MAKES SIX (1-CUP) SERVINGS

1/2 cup finely chopped onion
1/2 teaspoon minced garlic
1 (15-ounce) can solid pack pumpkin
3 1/2 cups canned fat-free chicken broth or
  vegetable broth
1/2 cup skim milk
Salt and pepper to taste
Nonfat plain yogurt

In a pot coated with nonstick cooking spray, sauté the onion and garlic over a medium heat until tender, about 5 minutes. Add the pumpkin. Gradually add the chicken broth and milk. Season with salt and pepper. Cook until heated through, about 5 minutes. Serve with a dollop of yogurt.

Nutritional information per serving
*Calories 45, Protein (g) 4, Carbohydrate (g) 8,
Fat (g) 0, Cal. from Fat (%) 0, Saturated Fat (g) 0,
Dietary Fiber (g) 3, Cholesterol (mg) 0, Sodium (mg) 391,
Diabetic Exchanges: 0.5 starch*

DOC'S NOTES:

Onions provide Vitamin C and folacin while the pumpkin provides beta carotene and Vitamin C.

Cheese Broccoli Soup 🥕 ❄

Broccoli is disguised in this nutritious creamy cheesy soup.

MAKES 6 TO 8 SERVINGS

2 tablespoons margarine

1 onion, chopped

1/2 cup all-purpose flour

3 cups canned fat-free chicken broth or
    vegetable broth

2 (10-ounce) packages frozen chopped broccoli,
    thawed and drained

1½ cups skim milk

4 ounces light pasteurized processed cheese
    spread, cut into cubes

Salt and pepper to taste

In a large saucepan, melt the margarine and sauté the onion until tender, about 5 minutes. Blend in the flour, stirring. Gradually add the chicken broth and then the broccoli, stirring to combine. Bring the mixture to a boil, stirring. Reduce heat to low. Cover and cook for 15 to 20 minutes or until the broccoli is done and the soup thickens. Add the milk, stirring until blended. Add the cheese cubes to the soup, stirring and cooking over a low heat until the cheese is melted and smooth. Season to taste. If you want a cheesier soup, just add extra cheese.

Nutritional information per serving
Calories 135, Protein (g) 9, Carbohydrate (g) 16, Fat (g) 5, Cal. from Fat (%) 30, Saturated Fat (g) 2, Dietary Fiber (g) 3, Cholesterol (mg) 7, Sodium (mg) 527, Diabetic Exchanges: 0.5 lean meat, 0.5 starch, 1 vegetable, 1 fat

DOC'S NOTES:

This soup is hearty and healthy. Broccoli is not only a good source of Vitamin C and beta carotene, it also contains nitrogen compounds called indoles, which may be protective against certain forms of cancer. As long as the veggies are cooked, enjoy!

Two-Potato Bisque ❄

*Here's a different and delicious twist
on bisque.*

Makes 4 to 6 serving

1 large sweet potato (yam), peeled and
  cut into 1-inch cubes
1 large baking potato, peeled and
  cut into 1-inch cubes
1 onion, chopped
2 cloves garlic, minced
1 bay leaf
Salt to taste
1 teaspoon dried thyme leaves
2 cups canned fat-free chicken broth
1 cup buttermilk
1 cup skim milk
2 tablespoons lime juice

In a large pot, combine the sweet potato, baking potato, onion, garlic, bay leaf, salt, thyme, and chicken broth and bring to a boil. Reduce the heat and simmer, covered, for 15 minutes, or until the potatoes are tender. Pour the mixture into a food processor and blend until smooth; return to the pot. Add the buttermilk, skim milk, and lime juice and cook over a low heat just until heated through; do not boil. Remove bay leaf before serving.

Nutritional information per serving

*Calories 100, Protein (g) 6, Carbohydrate (g) 20,
Fat (g) 0, Cal. from Fat (%) 0, Saturated Fat (g) 0,
Dietary Fiber (g) 2, Cholesterol (mg) 0, Sodium (mg) 281,
Diabetic Exchanges: 1 starch, 0.5 skim milk*

DOC'S NOTES:

The baking potato provides a good source of protein, complex carbohydrates and potassium whit the sweet potato is a good source of beta carotene, fiber, and vitamins B and C.

Artichoke Soup

A few cans thrown in the food processor makes a wonderful creamy creation.

MAKES 6 TO 8 SERVINGS

3 (14-ounce) cans artichoke hearts, drained
3 (10¾-ounce) cans fat-free cream of
   mushroom soup
1 cup skim milk
2 cups canned fat-free chicken broth or
   vegetable broth
½ cup dry white wine, optional

Place artichokes in a food processor and purÄe. Combine remaining ingredients in a bowl and add to processor. Blend until well combined. Transfer to a pot and heat over low heat to serve.

Nutritional information per serving

Calories 112, Protein (g) 5, Carbohydrate (g) 17,
Fat (g) 3, Cal. from Fat (%) 23, Saturated Fat (g) 1,
Dietary Fiber (g) 1, Cholesterol (mg) 5, Sodium (mg) 1200,
Diabetic Exchanges: 0.5 starch, 0.5 vegetable, 0.5 fat

DOC'S NOTES:

This can be served at room temperature. Artichokes are high in Vitamin C, folacin, magnesium, phosphorus, and potassium. Artichokes offer a health protective substance called silymarin, which may play a role in cancer prevention.

Easy Crab Soup ❄

A quick version when in a pinch!

MAKES 4 SERVINGS

1 onion, finely chopped

2 tablespoons margarine

2 tablespoons all-purpose flour

1³/₄ cups canned fat-free chicken broth

¹/₂ cup water

1 (12-ounce) can evaporated skimmed milk

1 pound lump or white crabmeat, picked for bones

3 green onion stems (scallions), finely
chopped, optional

In a saucepan, sauté onion in margarine until tender. Stir in flour and gradually add broth and water. Simmer for 20 minutes on low heat. Stir in milk. Fold in crabmeat. Garnish with green onion stems when not neutropenic.

Nutritional information per serving

Calories 286, Protein (g) 35, Carbohydrate (g) 19, Fat (g) 7, Cal. from Fat (%) 23, Saturated Fat (g) 1, Dietary Fiber (g) 1, Cholesterol (mg) 90, Sodium (mg) 888, Diabetic Exchanges: 4 very lean meat, 1 skim milk, 1 vegetable, 1 fat

DOC'S NOTES:

Use green onion as a garnish only when not neutropenic.

Linguine
Florentine 🥕 ❄️

Spinach and linguine combine together for a light but satisfying meal. Serve smaller portions as a side to any entrée.

MAKES 6 SERVINGS

2 tablespoons olive oil

1 teaspoon minced garlic

1 large bunch fresh spinach, (5 to 6 cups), stemmed and washed

1 (12-ounce) can evaporated skimmed milk

Salt and pepper to taste

1 (16-ounce) package linguine

1/3 cup grated Parmesan cheese

In a large skillet, heat the oil and add the garlic and spinach. Cover and cook until the spinach is wilted, about 3 minutes, stirring occasionally. Add the milk and season to taste. Meanwhile, prepare the pasta according to package directions; drain. Toss with the spinach in the skillet and sprinkle with the cheese.

Nutritional information per serving

Calories 402, Protein (g) 18, Carbohydrate (g) 65, Fat (g) 8, Cal. from Fat (%) 17, Saturated Fat (g) 2, Dietary Fiber (g) 3, Cholesterol (mg) 7, Sodium (mg) 202, Diabetic Exchanges: 4 starch, 0.5 skim milk, 1 fat

DOC'S NOTES:

Cooked veggies are fine when white blood cell count is low.

Loaded Potatoes

These yummy potatoes can be served plain or add your favorite condiments depending on your taste tolerance.

MAKES 6 SERVINGS

1 (32-ounce) bag frozen hash brown potatoes
2 large eggs
3 large egg whites
2 cups skim milk
4 tablespoons margarine, melted
Salt and pepper to taste
1/2 teaspoon onion powder
2 cups shredded reduced-fat Cheddar cheese
1/2 cup nonfat plain yogurt
1/2 cup salsa, optional

Preheat oven to 350 degrees. Place the potatoes in a 1 1/2-quart shallow baking dish coated with nonstick cooking spray. Bake for 15 minutes. Meanwhile, combine the eggs, egg whites, milk, margarine, salt and pepper, and onion powder. Remove the potatoes from the oven. Sprinkle with the Cheddar cheese, tossing toss with a fork to mix. Pour the milk mixture over the potatoes. Return to the oven and bake for 30 to 40 minutes longer or until the potatoes are light brown and firm to touch. Serve with salsa.

Nutritional information per serving

Calories 379, Protein (g) 22, Carbohydrate (g) 34, Fat (g) 17, Cal. from Fat (%) 41, Saturated Fat (g) 7, Dietary Fiber (g) 2, Cholesterol (mg) 93, Sodium (mg) 561, Diabetic Exchanges: 2 lean meat, 2 starch, 0.5 skim milk, 2 fat

DOC'S NOTES:

If neutropenic, don't use salsa or green onions.

Cheesy Shrimp Rice Casserole

A palate pleasing plain recipe.

MAKES 6 TO 8 SERVINGS

1 cup dry brown or wild rice

2 cups water

2 pounds cooked medium shrimp, peeled

Salt and pepper to taste

6 ounces light pasteurized processed
   cheese spread

1/2 cup skim milk

Bread crumbs

Preheat oven to 350 degrees. Cook the rice in the water according to package directions. Set aside. Combine the shrimp, salt and pepper, and the cooked rice. Heat the cheese and milk together in the microwave or in a small pan over medium-low heat until melted, and mix with the rice mixture. Transfer to a 2-quart casserole dish, sprinkle with bread crumbs, and bake for 15 minutes or until well heated.

Nutritional information per serving

Calories 250, Protein (g) 30, Carbohydrate (g) 21, Fat (g) 4, Cal. from Fat (%) 15, Saturated Fat (g) 2, Dietary Fiber (g) 1, Cholesterol (mg) 230, Sodium (mg) 601, Diabetic Exchanges: 5 very lean meat, 1.5 starch

DOC'S NOTES:

A single salad and this casserole is a complete meal. For sore mouth, finely chop shrimp.

Chicken Pot Pie ❄

I always get excited when I prepare this recipe, because it looks just as perfect as the commercially prepared ones but it tastes so much better! Use leftover chicken.

MAKES 6 SERVINGS

1 cup diced carrot

1 cup sliced mushrooms

1/2 cup chopped celery

1/2 cup frozen peas, thawed

1/4 cup finely chopped onion

1/4 cup all-purpose flour

1 (12-ounce) can evaporated skimmed milk

2 cups diced cooked skinless, boneless
  chicken breasts

1/2 teaspoon pepper, optional

1/2 teaspoon dried thyme leaves

1 cup self-rising flour

1 tablespoon canola oil

1/2 cup skim milk

Preheat oven to 450 degrees. Coat a large skillet with nonstick cooking spray and place over medium-high heat. Add the carrots, mushrooms, celery, peas, and onion and sauté 5 minutes, or until the vegetables are tender. Stir in the all-purpose flour. Gradually add the evaporated milk, stirring until the mixture thickens. Stir in the chicken, pepper, and thyme. Transfer the mixture into a 9-inch pie plate coated with nonstick cooking spray. Place the self-rising flour in a small bowl; cut in the oil with a pastry blender or two knives until the mixture is crumbly. Gradually add milk, stirring just until the ingredients are moistened. Drop the dough evenly by spoonfuls onto the chicken mixture. Bake, uncovered, for 15 to 20 minutes, or until the crust is golden.

Nutritional information per serving

Calories 273, Protein (g) 24, Carbohydrate (g) 33, Fat (g) 5, Cal. from Fat (%) 15, Saturated Fat (g) 1, Dietary Fiber (g) 2, Cholesterol (mg) 42, Sodium (mg) 414, Diabetic Exchanges: 2 very lean meat, 1.5 starch, 0.5 skim milk, 1 vegetable

DOC'S NOTES:

This is a complete meal. Carrots provide beta carotene and fiber while the mushrooms are filled with B vitamins, copper, and other minerals. Celery is rich in Vitamin C and folacin.

Chicken Piccata ❄

This recipe continually gets rave reviews in my house. Simple elegance.

MAKES 6 TO 8 SERVINGS

½ cup all-purpose flour
Salt and pepper to taste
1 teaspoon dried oregano leaves
2 pounds boneless skinless chicken breasts
3 tablespoons olive oil
2 cups canned fat-free chicken broth
1 teaspoon minced garlic
¼ cup lemon juice
2 tablespoons chopped parsley, optional

In a small bowl, combine flour, salt and pepper, and oregano. Coat each chicken piece with mixture; set aside. In a skillet coated with nonstick cooking spray, heat oil and cook chicken breasts on each side until golden brown over medium-high heat. Remove chicken from pan as needed to brown all pieces. Add chicken broth, garlic, and lemon juice to pan, scraping sides of pan. Return chicken to pan and bring to a boil. Reduce heat, cover, and simmer for 10 to 15 minutes or until chicken is done. Sprinkle with parsley, if not neutropenic, and serve.

Nutritional information per serving
Calories 205, Protein (g) 28, Carbohydrate (g) 7,
Fat (g) 7, Cal. from Fat (%) 30, Saturated Fat (g) 1,
Dietary Fiber (g) 0, Cholesterol (mg) 66, Sodium (mg) 229,
Diabetic Exchanges: 3 very lean meat, 0.5 starch, 1 fat

DOC'S NOTES:

Don't use fresh parsley if neutropenic.

Very Good Veal ❄

Veal is a nice variation from time to time.

MAKES 6 SERVINGS

1½ pounds thinly sliced veal (scaloppini)
¼ cup all-purpose flour
1 tablespoon paprika
Salt and pepper to taste
1 tablespoon margarine
½ teaspoon minced garlic
¼ cup water
1 cup nonfat plain yogurt
1 teaspoon dried basil leaves
1 tablespoon lemon juice
½ teaspoon dried rosemary leaves
¼ cup Marsala wine, optional

Cut the veal into bite-size pieces. Combine the flour, paprika, and salt and pepper in a plastic zip-top bag. Drop the veal into the bag and shake to coat well. In a large skillet, melt the margarine and add the veal pieces and garlic. Sauté over a medium high heat about 3 minutes, turning frequently, until the veal is browned. Add the water, scraping the bottom of the skillet. Lower the heat and stir in the yogurt, one spoonful at a time until well blended. Mix in the basil, lemon juice, rosemary, and Marsala wine. Heat thoroughly, about 5 minutes, but do not boil.

Nutritional information per serving
Calories 192, Protein (g) 25, Carbohydrate (g) 8, Fat (g) 6, Cal. from Fat (%) 28, Saturated Fat (g) 2, Dietary Fiber (g) 1, Cholesterol (mg) 103, Sodium (mg) 164, Diabetic Exchanges: 3 lean meat, 0.5 starch

DOC'S NOTES:

This is easy to prepare and is a good meal for a special occasion such as the night before your last chemotherapy treatment.

NEUTROPENIA

Hot Fruit Compote

Open cans and you have a tasty fruit dish. Great substitute for fresh fruit.

MAKES 12 TO 15 SERVINGS

2 bananas, sliced
1 tablespoon lemon juice
1 (29-ounce) can "lite" sliced peaches, drained
1 (16-ounce) can "lite" pear halves,
    drained and sliced
1 (16-ounce) can "lite" apricot halves, drained
    and sliced
1 (16½-ounce) can pitted Bing cherries, drained
1 (20-ounce) can pineapple chunks in its own
    juice, drained
¼ cup cornstarch
1 cup light brown sugar
½ teaspoon curry
6 tablespoons margarine, melted

Preheat oven to 350 degrees. Sprinkle bananas with lemon juice. Mix peaches, pears, apricots, cherries, and pineapple with bananas. Transfer to a 3-quart glass baking dish. In small bowl, combine cornstarch, brown sugar, and curry. Sprinkle over fruit. Drizzle margarine over top of dish. Bake, covered, for 30 minutes. Uncover, and bake for another 15 minutes or until bubbly.

Nutritional information per serving
Calories 188, Protein (g) 1, Carbohydrate (g) 38,
Fat (g) 5, Cal. from Fat (%) 21, Saturated Fat (g) 1,
Dietary Fiber (g) 2, Cholesterol (mg) 0, Sodium (mg) 66,
Diabetic Exchanges: 1.5 fruit, 1 other carb., 1 fat

DOC'S NOTES:

This is a great source of fruit when you are neutropenic and cannot have fresh fruit. The fruits provide Vitamins A and C and beta carotene.

Heavenly Yam Delight 🥕

A sweet potato version of a favorite layered dessert. The perfect treat to make when you're in a hurry, wonderful! If you enjoy pumpkin, you'll love this treat.

MAKES 16 SERVINGS

1 cup all-purpose flour
1/4 cup plus 2/3 cup confectioners' sugar, divided
1/3 cup chopped pecans
6 tablespoons margarine, softened
1 (8-ounce) package fat-free cream cheese
1 (8-ounce) container fat-free frozen whipped topping, thawed, divided
1 (29-ounce) can sweet potatoes (yams), drained
1/2 teaspoon ground cinnamon
1/4 cup sugar

Preheat oven to 350 degrees. In a large bowl, combine flour, 1/4 cup confectioners' sugar, pecans, and margarine. Press into bottom of 13×9×2-inch baking pan. Bake 20 minutes. Set aside to cool. In a mixing bowl, mix cream cheese and remaining 2/3 cup confectioners' sugar until creamy. Fold in 3/4 cup whipped topping. Spread cream cheese mixture over cooled crust. In a mixing bowl, beat sweet potatoes, cinnamon, and sugar until smooth. Spread over cream cheese mixture. Top with remaining whipped topping. Refrigerate.

Nutritional information per serving

Calories 205, Protein (g) 4, Carbohydrate (g) 33, Fat (g) 6, Cal. from Fat (%) 28, Saturated Fat (g) 1, Dietary Fiber (g) 2, Cholesterol (mg) 1, Sodium (mg) 143, Diabetic Exchanges: 1 starch, 1 other carb., 1 fat

DOC'S NOTES:

When your white blood cell count is low, this will surely give you a lift. Remember your blood counts will normally only stay down for 4 to 7 days.

Mocha Cappuccino Pudding Pie 🥕 ❄

Sugar-free instant pudding and sugar-free ice cream may be substituted.

MAKES 8 SERVINGS

1 (4-serving) package instant chocolate pudding
2 teaspoons coffee granules
1 cup skim milk
1 cup fat-free vanilla ice cream
1 cup fat-free frozen whipped topping, thawed
1 prepared reduced-fat graham cracker crust

Combine pudding mix, coffee granules, milk, and ice cream. Beat 2 minutes or until creamy. Fold in whipped topping. Transfer to prepared pie crust. Freeze 30 minutes or longer before serving. Can also be made as a parfait.

Nutritional information per serving

Calories 203, Protein (g) 3, Carbohydrate (g) 39, Fat (g) 3, Cal. from Fat (%) 15, Saturated Fat (g) 1, Dietary Fiber (g) 1, Cholesterol (mg) 1, Sodium (mg) 332, Diabetic Exchanges: 1.5 starch, 1 other carb., 0.5 fat

DOC'S NOTES:

This is a great snack or use it as a dessert. Substitute a vanilla nutritional energy drink supplement for the skim milk to add vitamins, minerals, and calories.

Baked Peach Delight

This will intrigue your guests. A great substitute for fresh fruit. Adjust recipe according to number of peach halves in the can.

MAKES 5 SERVINGS

1 (16-ounce) can peach halves, drained
  (5 halves)
5 tablespoons reduced-fat peanut butter
5 teaspoons light brown sugar

Preheat oven to 350 degrees. Place peach halves in a baking dish, pit-side up. Spread 1 tablespoon peanut butter on each peach half and sprinkle each with 1 teaspoon brown sugar. Bake until peanut butter and brown sugar melt, about 5 to 10 minutes.

Nutritional information per serving

Calories 135, Protein (g) 5, Carbohydrate (g) 20, Fat (g) 5, Cal. from Fat (%) 33, Saturated Fat (g) 1, Dietary Fiber (g) 2, Cholesterol (mg) 0, Sodium (mg) 94, Diabetic Exchanges: 0.5 very lean meat, 1 fruit, 0.5 other carb., 1 fat

DOC'S NOTES:

Peaches provide the Vitamin C while the peanut butter adds protein to this dish.

Peach Smoothie 🥕

Serve with gingersnaps or honey graham crackers.

MAKES TWO (1-CUP) SERVINGS

2 cups canned sliced peaches, drained
1 (12-ounce) can peach nectar
1 cup nonfat vanilla yogurt
1/2 teaspoon almond extract, optional
1 cup chopped ice

In a food processor or blender, combine all ingredients and blend until mixture is smooth and frothy.

Nutritional information per serving

Calories 326, Protein (g) 8, Carbohydrate (g) 77, Fat (g) 0, Cal. from Fat (%) 0, Saturated Fat (g) 0, Dietary Fiber (g) 4, Cholesterol (mg) 0, Sodium (mg) 107, Diabetic Exchanges: 3 fruit, 1 skim milk, 1 other carb.

DOC'S NOTES:

For extra vitamins and calories, use a nutritional energy drink supplement instead of the yogurt.

Peach Weight Gain Shake 🥕

Peaches and almond disguise the taste of the supplement.

MAKES 2 SERVINGS

1 (12-ounce) can vanilla nutritional energy
  drink supplement
1/2 teaspoon almond extract
1 (15-ounce) can sliced peaches in syrup, drained

Pour supplement, extract, and peaches into a blender. Blend and chill or serve over ice.

Nutritional information per serving

Calories 298, Protein (g) 8, Carbohydrate (g) 61, Fat (g) 3, Cal. from Fat (%) 9, Saturated Fat (g) 0, Dietary Fiber (g) 2, Cholesterol (mg) 0, Sodium (mg) 106, Diabetic Exchanges: 2 starch, 2 fruit

DOC'S NOTES:

Remember to have an adequate number of calories per day.

Basic Weight Gain Shake 🥕

Also great for sore mouth. Add frozen banana if desired.

MAKES 1 SERVING

½ cup chocolate nutritional energy drink
  supplement, chilled
½ cup reduced-fat vanilla ice cream

Place supplement and ice cream in a blender and blend until well mixed. Pour into a large glass and serve.

Nutritional information per serving

Calories 228, Protein (g) 8, Carbohydrate (g) 39, Fat (g) 4, Cal. from Fat (%) 16, Saturated Fat (g) 1, Dietary Fiber (g) 1, Cholesterol (mg) 5, Sodium (mg) 109, Diabetic Exchanges: 0.5 very lean meat, 1.5 starch, 1 other carb., 0.5 fat

DOC'S NOTES:

Great supplement for extra calories as it includes all the vitamins and nutrients you need to survive.

Hot Cocoa Drink Supplement 🥕

Packages of cocoa mix turn these drinks into chocolate delights. Coffee lovers, stir in 1/2 teaspoon instant coffee. For Cocoa Smoothie, add cocoa mix to 1/2 cup chilled chocolate nutritional energy drink supplement and 1/2 cup ice cubes in a blender and blend until smooth.

MAKES 1 SERVING

1 (8-ounce) can nutritional energy
  drink supplement
1 package hot cocoa mix

Pour supplement into a large microwave-safe mug and microwave until very hot. Gradually stir in the cocoa mix until well blended.

Nutritional information per serving

Calories 348, Protein (g) 11, Carbohydrate (g) 65, Fat (g) 5, Cal. from Fat (%) 13, Saturated Fat (g) 0, Dietary Fiber (g) 1, Cholesterol (mg) 2, Sodium (mg) 230, Diabetic Exchanges: 0.5 very lean meat, 3 starch, 1.5 other carb.

DOC'S NOTES:

A great drink on cold mornings for extra calories, vitamins, and minerals.

Diarrhea

- Will it ever stop?
- Should I stop eating and drinking altogether?
- What should I eat and drink?
- Is it alright to take Immodium, Lomotil or Pepto Bismol?
- My rectum is sore, what can I do? (Don't panic, help is on the way!)

Diarrhea can follow certain chemotherapy or radiation treatments. This can be a problem with certain drugs such as 5-FU, CPT-11 and antibiotics. If the diarrhea starts, the first thing to do is to stop all intake of high fiber foods—such as nuts, seeds, whole grains, legumes, dried fruit and raw fruits and vegetables—stool softeners or laxatives. Follow your doctors' instructions with regards to Lomotil, Immodium, or Pepto Bismol. Start clear liquids after fasting two to four hours. Force fluids up to eight to ten glasses per day. Water, clear soup, broth, flat soda or a sports drink are excellent fluids to replace those lost by diarrhea. Avoid dairy products since they tend to make diarrhea worse. Avoid gassy foods and carbonated beverages. Hot and cold beverages, alcohol, coffee and cigarettes tend to aggravate diarrhea. Be sure to sip fluids throughout the day to prevent dehydration.

Bananas, rice, applesauce and toast are good foods to begin eating following a decrease in your diarrhea. Once you are tolerating these foods, progress to bland low fiber foods, such as chicken without the skin, scrambled eggs, and canned or cooked fruits without skins. Crackers, pasta without sauce, white bread or gelatins are good choices. Try to avoid foods high in fiber, such as grains, raw vegetables, whole wheat, raw fruit, oatmeal and brown rice.

Nuts, beans and milk products may worsen the diarrhea. Any high fat food should be avoided. Try to avoid caffeine and hot or spicy foods. Once your diarrhea has subsided, you can adjust your diet accordingly. Foods low in fiber and fat are helpful in decreasing your diarrhea.

If your rectum becomes red or sore, use a commercial wet towel without alcohol and avoid dry toilet paper. Desitin or a combination of Aquaphor and Questran in a 9 to 1 ratio, will act as a protective barrier to your perirectal area. Ask your physician to prescribe these medications.

If your diarrhea continues without relief for greater than twenty-four hours, please notify your physician. I hope the recipes and suggestions that follow will help to get you regulated and eating healthy again.

Points to Remember

- ✦ Eat chicken soup or bouillon cubes dissolved in water.
- ✦ Eat bland, high-protein foods.
- ✦ Eat smaller mini meals throughout the day to see what you can tolerate.
- ✦ Eat high-calorie, low-fiber foods.
- ✦ Avoid citrus juices and carbonated beverages. An alternative to carbonated drinks is mineral water with a splash of fruit juices, which is both bubbly and tasty.
- ✦ Avoid raw vegetables and fruits, and high fiber foods, nuts, onions, garlic, and gaseous vegetables.
- ✦ Avoid spicy foods.
- ✦ Avoid greasy, fatty, or fried foods.
- ✦ Drink beverages frequently, in small amounts, and at room temperatures.
- ✦ Limit caffeine intake.
- ✦ Choose low fiber light foods like fish, chicken, eggs, bananas, potatoes, low fiber cereals, crackers, refined bread and flour products. Crackers with peanut butter or cheese sometimes works.
- ✦ Do minimal activity after meals.
- ✦ Ginger can be soothing to the stomach: gingersnaps, ginger candy
- ✦ Drink plenty of mild, clear, non-carbonated liquids throughout the day. Drink liquids at room temperature, as they are better tolerated than hot or cold beverages. Flat soda is another good choice.
- ✦ Limit milk.
- ✦ Avoid drinks and foods that cause gas, such as carbonated drinks, chewing gum and gas-forming vegetables (broccoli, cauliflower, cabbage, Brussels sprouts and beans). Drink carbonated beverages if you leave them open for at least 10 minutes before drinking
- ✦ Drink and eat high-sodium foods such as broths, soups, sports drinks, crackers, baked chips and pretzels.
- ✦ Drink and eat high-potassium foods such as fruit juices and nectars, sports drinks, potatoes without the skin, and bananas.
- ✦ Eat foods high in pectin such as applesauce and bananas.

- Avoid chewing gums, sugar-free gums, and all candies made with sorbitol.
- Be sure to sip fluids throughout the day to prevent dehydration.
- When recommended by a healthcare practitioner, soluble fiber can be used to relieve mild to moderate diarrhea. Soluble fiber soaks up a significant amount of water in the digestive tract causing stool to be more firm and pass slower. *Soluble fiber sources include:* Legumes, oats, bananas, apples, berries, broccoli, carrots, potatoes and yams (without skins).

Some Foods to Include
- Toast, crackers or pretzels
- Flavored gelatin
- Applesauce
- Skinless chicken
- Clear liquids
- Bananas
- Rice
- Plums, peaches, watermelon, cantaloupe
- Squash, eggplant

When You Are Feeling Queasy
If you experience nausea and vomiting, try to drink fluids to prevent dehydration. Sip water, juices, and other clear, calorie-containing liquids throughout the day. You may tolerate clear, cool liquids better than very hot or icy fluids. When you have stopped vomiting, try eating easy-to-digest foods such as clear liquids, crackers, gelatin, and plain toast.

Points to Remember
- Eat six to eight small meals a day, instead of three large meals.
- Eat dry foods, such as crackers, toast, dry cereals, pretzels or bread sticks, when you wake up and every few hours during the day.
- Eat foods that do not have a strong odor.
- Eat cool foods instead of hot spicy foods.

- ✦ Avoid foods that are overly sweet, greasy, fried, or spicy, such as rich desserts and French fries.
- ✦ Sit up or recline with your head raised for at least 1 hour after eating if you need to rest.
- ✦ Sip clear liquids frequently to prevent dehydration.
- ✦ Ask your doctor about medications that prevent or stop nausea.
- ✦ Try bland, soft, easy-to-digest foods on scheduled treatment days. Foods such as cream of wheat and chicken noodle soup with saltine crackers may be better tolerated than heavy meals.
- ✦ Avoid eating in a room that is warm, or that has cooking odors or other smells. Cook outside on the grill or use boiling bags to reduce cooking odors.
- ✦ Rinse your mouth before and after meals.
- ✦ Suck on hard candy, such as peppermint or lemon, if there is a bad taste in your mouth.
- ✦ Drink eight or more cups of liquid each day if you can. Drink an additional half cup to one cup of liquid for each episode of vomiting. Try sipping liquids 30 to 60 minutes after eating solid food.
- ✦ Ginger is an herb recognized to help with nausea. Try drinking ginger tea or flat ginger ale.

Shopping List for Diarrhea
- ✦ Bananas
- ✦ Bread
- ✦ Skinless boneless chicken breasts
- ✦ Cheese
- ✦ Clear liquids
- ✦ Energy drinks
- ✦ Nutritional energy drink supplement
- ✦ Pasta
- ✦ Roasted turkey breast
- ✦ Rice
- ✦ Squash

Menus

Foods to eat to ease diarrhea.

Breakfast

Scrambled Eggs

Grits

80   Easy Banana Bread

25   Baked French Toast

22   Cinnamon Rolls

Lunch

85   Quick Chicken Pasta

Applesauce

Rolls

Plain Turkey Sandwich

Dinner

Oven Fried Parmesan Chicken   84

Baked Potato

Banana Pudding   87

Chicken Scampi   86

Pasta

Mocha Meringue Mounds   198

Roasted Turkey Breast   83

Pasta Toss   82

Coffee Cake   196

Snacks

Banana Bread   174

Cinnamon Quick Bread   156

Banana Puff   81

Easy Banana Bread ✎ ❄

This is a short cut banana bread, thanks to the biscuit mix.

MAKES 16 SLICES

1 (8-ounce) package reduced-fat
  cream cheese, softened
1 cup sugar
3 medium bananas, mashed
1 large egg, beaten
2 large egg whites
2 cups biscuit baking mix
1/2 teaspoon ground cinnamon

Preheat oven to 350 degrees. Coat a 9×5×3-inch loaf pan with nonstick cooking spray. In a mixing bowl, cream together the cream cheese and sugar until light. Beat in the bananas, egg, and egg whites. Stir in the biscuit mix and cinnamon until just blended. Turn into the prepared loaf pan. Bake for 45 minutes to 1 hour, until a toothpick inserted in the center comes out clean. Cool in the pan 15 minutes.

Nutritional information per serving
*Calories 168, Protein (g) 3, Carbohydrate (g) 28,
Fat (g) 5, Cal. from Fat (%) 26, Saturated Fat (g) 2,
Dietary Fiber (g) 1, Cholesterol (mg) 20, Sodium (mg) 267,
Diabetic Exchanges: 0.5 starch, 0.5 fruit, 1 other carb.,
0.5 fat*

DOC'S NOTES:

Bananas are a great source of potassium. They are easily digested by virtually everyone. The high carbohydrate content makes bananas the snack of choice for endurance athletes.

Banana Puff 🥕 ❄️

A light tasty meal for breakfast or any time of day.

MAKES 8 SERVINGS

2 eggs, separated
1/4 cup sugar
1 cup nonfat plain yogurt
2 tablespoons margarine, melted
1 teaspoon vanilla extract
1/2 teaspoon imitation butter flavoring
3/4 cup all-purpose flour
2 teaspoons baking powder
1 teaspoon baking soda
1/4 teaspoon ground cinnamon
1 banana, diced

Preheat oven to 400 degrees. In a mixing bowl, beat egg yolks, sugar, yogurt, and margarine until blended. Add flavorings. Combine dry ingredients, and beat into egg mixture until all ingredients are moistened. In another bowl, beat egg whites until stiff. Carefully fold into batter. Fold in bananas. Spread batter into a 9-inch round cake pan coated with nonstick cooking spray. Bake for 20 to 25 minutes. Serve immediately.

Nutritional information per serving

Calories 145, Protein (g) 5, Carbohydrate (g) 22, Fat (g) 4, Cal. from Fat (%) 27, Saturated Fat (g) 1, Dietary Fiber (g) 1, Cholesterol (mg) 54, Sodium (mg) 352, Diabetic Exchanges: 0.5 starch, 0.5 fruit, 0.5 other carb., 1 fat

Pasta Toss 🥕

DIARRHEA

Use whatever pasta that is in your pantry.

MAKES 8 SERVINGS

1 (16-ounce) package pasta
2 tablespoons olive oil
1 cup chopped tomato
1 tablespoon minced garlic
1 teaspoon dried basil leaves
1 cup coarsely chopped green onions (scallions)
1/3 cup grated Parmesan cheese

Prepare the pasta according to package directions; drain and set aside. In a large skillet, heat the olive oil and sauté tomato and garlic for 1 minute. Add the basil and green onions and pasta. Toss with the Parmesan cheese.

Nutritional information per serving

Calories 270, Protein (g) 10, Carbohydrate (g) 45, Fat (g) 6, Cal. from Fat (%) 19, Saturated Fat (g) 1, Dietary Fiber (g) 2, Cholesterol (mg) 3, Sodium (mg) 86, Diabetic Exchanges: 3 starch, 1 fat

DOC'S NOTES:

Depending on how you feel, adjust the amount of tomatoes and green onions.

Roasted Turkey Breast ❄

Easy and herbs enhance a plain turkey breast.

MAKES 8 SERVINGS

1 (3-pound) fresh turkey breast
1/2 cup canned fat-free chicken broth
1 tablespoon dried rosemary leaves
1 teaspoon garlic powder
1 teaspoon dried thyme leaves
1 teaspoon dried oregano leaves
1/4 teaspoon black pepper

Preheat oven to 375 degrees. Rinse the breast and pat dry. Place in a shallow baking dish. Add the broth and enough water to come up to 1/4 inch in the dish. Sprinkle the rosemary, garlic powder, thyme, oregano, and pepper all over turkey. Bake for 1 to 1 1/2 hours or until the internal temperature is 170 degrees on a meat thermometer. Remove skin before serving.

Nutritional information per serving
Calories 150, Protein (g) 33, Carbohydrate (g) 1, Fat (g) 1, Cal. from Fat (%) 6, Saturated Fat (g) 0, Dietary Fiber (g) 0, Cholesterol (mg) 89, Sodium (mg) 119, Diabetic Exchanges: 4 very lean meat

DOC'S NOTES:

Light and easy on the stomach when you have had problems with diarrhea.

Oven Fried Parmesan Chicken ❄

Easy, tasty and will fulfill your urge for old-fashioned fried chicken. Cut recipe in half to prepare less. This chicken is good the next day on a sandwich.

MAKES 10 SERVINGS

3/4 cup nonfat plain yogurt
1/4 cup lemon juice
1 1/2 tablespoons Dijon mustard
3 cloves garlic, minced
1/2 teaspoon dried oregano leaves
10 boneless, skinless chicken breasts
2 tablespoons margarine, melted

Combine all ingredients except margarine. Marinate, covered, 2 hours or overnight in refrigerator. Preheat oven to 350 degrees. Drain chicken and coat with Bread Crumb Coating (recipe follows). Place on a baking sheet coated with nonstick cooking spray and chill for 1 hour (if time permits). Drizzle chicken with margarine. Bake for 45 minutes to 1 hour or until tender and golden brown.

BREAD CRUMB COATING

2 cups dry bread crumbs or Italian bread crumbs
1/4 cup grated Parmesan cheese

Combine all coating ingredients in shallow bowl.

Nutritional information per serving
Calories 246, Protein (g) 30, Carbohydrate (g) 16, Fat (g) 6, Cal. from Fat (%) 21, Saturated Fat (g) 2, Dietary Fiber (g) 1, Cholesterol (mg) 68, Sodium (mg) 347, Diabetic Exchanges: 3 lean meat, 1 starch

Quick Chicken Pasta ❄

When feeling better, this dish is quick to prepare and quick to disappear from the plate. If you can't tolerate mushrooms, onion or tomato, leave out for a plainer version, until you feel better.

MAKES 4 SERVINGS

1 tablespoon olive oil

2 pounds boneless skinless chicken breasts, cut into strips

Salt and pepper to taste

1 large tomato, diced, optional

1 cup sliced mushrooms, optional

1 teaspoon minced garlic

1/2 cup chopped red onion, optional

1 tablespoon dried basil leaves

1/3 cup canned fat-free chicken broth

1 (8-ounce) package angel hair (capellini) pasta

1/4 cup grated Romano cheese

In a large pan coated with nonstick cooking spray, heat the olive oil and sauté the chicken until almost done, about 4 minutes. Season with salt and pepper. Add the tomato, mushrooms, garlic, onion, and basil, stirring for 5 minutes or until veggies are tender. Add the chicken broth, cooking until heated through. Meanwhile, cook the pasta according to package directions, omitting any oil and salt. Drain and set aside. When the chicken is done, toss with the pasta and Romano cheese.

Nutritional information per serving

Calories 507, Protein (g) 61, Carbohydrate (g) 43, Fat (g) 8, Cal. from Fat (%) 15, Saturated Fat (g) 2, Dietary Fiber (g) 2, Cholesterol (mg) 134, Sodium (mg) 229, Diabetic Exchanges: 7 very lean meat, 3 starch

DOC'S NOTES:

Leaving out the onions and tomatoes will make this dish an excellent meal if you have diarrhea.

Chicken Scampi ❄

Cut the chicken into strips and toss with pasta and you have a super combination. I have always loved shrimp scampi and now you can enjoy the same flavor with chicken.

MAKES 6 SERVINGS

2 pounds boneless, skinless chicken breasts
1 tablespoon olive oil
2 tablespoons grated Parmesan cheese
1 tablespoon dried parsley flakes
1/4 teaspoon garlic powder
Salt and pepper to taste
1 tablespoon dried oregano leaves
3 tablespoons lemon juice
2 tablespoons Worcestershire sauce

Combine all the ingredients in a shallow bowl. Marinate, covered, in the refrigerator for several hours or overnight. Preheat the broiler. Remove the chicken from the marinade and place in a single layer in a shallow baking dish or broiling pan. Broil 8 inches from the heat, turning once, until the chicken is done, about 15 minutes.

Nutritional information per serving
Calories 176, Protein (g) 35, Carbohydrate (g) 1, Fat (g) 3, Cal. from Fat (%) 14, Saturated Fat (g) 1, Dietary Fiber (g) 0, Cholesterol (mg) 88, Sodium (mg) 146, Diabetic Exchanges: 4 very lean meat

DOC'S NOTES:

You will find this dish to be light and easy on your gastrointestinal tract. Boiled plain pasta and dry toast is a good meal to try once your diarrhea is decreasing.

Banana Pudding ✐

Layer with vanilla wafers and bananas for an old-fashioned banana pudding. Sugar-free pudding may be substituted.

MAKES 4 SERVINGS

1 (4-serving) package instant banana
  pudding mix
2 cups skim milk
2 bananas, diced

In a mixing bowl, mix banana pudding and milk with a whisk for 2 minutes. Fold cut up bananas into pudding. For pudding, transfer to cups and refrigerate.

Nutritional information per serving

*Calories 188, Protein (g) 5, Carbohydrate (g) 43,
Fat (g) 1, Cal. from Fat (%) 3, Saturated Fat (g) 0,
Dietary Fiber (g) 1, Cholesterol (mg) 2, Sodium (mg) 435,
Diabetic Exchanges: 0.5 skim milk, 1 fruit, 1.5 other carb.*

DOC'S NOTES:

For extra calories, substitute vanilla nutritional energy drink supplement for skim milk. It's a great way to sneak extra vitamins and calories into your diet. No bananas if your blood counts are low.

Glazed Bananas

Serve over frozen vanilla yogurt at a later date and you will have a sensational simple dessert.

MAKES 6 SERVINGS

2 tablespoons margarine
1/4 cup light brown sugar
1/8 teaspoon ground cinnamon
1/4 cup orange juice
3 firm bananas, peeled, split lengthwise
    and halved

In pan, heat margarine, brown sugar, cinnamon, and orange juice until bubbly. Add banana slices and cook for 5 minutes, turning as needed. Serve immediately.

Nutritional information per serving
Calories 127, Protein (g) 1, Carbohydrate (g) 24, Fat (g) 4, Cal. from Fat (%) 27, Saturated Fat (g) 1, Dietary Fiber (g) 2, Cholesterol (mg) 0, Sodium (mg) 49, Diabetic Exchanges: 1 fruit, 0.5 other carb., 1 fat

DOC'S NOTES:

This can be eaten with or without the yogurt. Great food if diarrhea is a problem. Bananas help to replace the potassium lost with the diarrhea.

DIARRHEA

Constipation

- ✦ How often do I need to have a bowel movement?
- ✦ Should I take a stool softener?
- ✦ Why am I constipated when I have never had this problem before?
- ✦ Are there any foods that will aid in the relief of my constipation?

Constipation can be a problem at any time during your treatment. Certain drugs such as pain medicines and chemotherapy, namely Vincristine, are commonly associated with constipation. Normally, you need to have a bowel movement every forty-eight to seventy-two hours. This will vary among people. You should only be concerned if you notice a difference from your normal routine.

Stool softeners such as Colace, Surfak, and Senokot are very helpful. Again, six to eight glasses of water is mandatory. Bulk forming agents such as Fibercon, Citrucel, or Metamucil will aid your constipation immensely. Laxatives including Milk of Magnesia, Ducolax, Lactulose, Mineral Oil, Magnesium Citrate, in addition to water and a stool softener or bulk forming agent, will alleviate your constipation.

Constipation will decrease your appetite and generally make you feel bad. Foods high in fiber, such as bran, should be a part of your everyday diet. Muffins made with prune juice instead of water can aid the problem. Fruit salads, vegetable dishes, beans, grains, dried fruit, seeds, raw fruits and vegetables, bread, fruit drinks, figs, raisins, apples, brown rice, pudding and stewed prunes are a few foods which can help keep you regular. If a healthy diet, stool softeners, and laxatives fail, contact your physician. You should not go over seventy-two hours without a bowel movement. The following foods and recipes should really be helpful for you. In addition, drink plenty of fluids throughout the day, eat at regular times, and increase your level of physical activity.

Points to Remember

- ✦ Drink 8 to 10 cups of liquid each day, if OK with your doctor. In addition to water, try fluids that have calories like prune juice, warm juices, teas, and hot lemonade.
- ✦ Limit drinks and foods that cause gas if it becomes a problem. These include carbonated drinks, broccoli, cabbage, cauliflower, cucumbers, dried beans, peas, and onions.
- ✦ Eat high-fiber and bulky foods, such as whole grain breads and cereals, fruits and vegetables (raw and cooked with skins and peels on), popcorn, and dried beans.
- ✦ Eat a breakfast that includes a hot drink and high-fiber foods.
- ✦ Increase intake of high-fiber foods.
- ✦ Try adding shredded veggies into other casseroles or recipes.
- ✦ Add oat or wheat bran to casseroles.
- ✦ Try adding 2 tablespoons wheat bran a day to your diet…drink water.
- ✦ Bran such as wheat bran may be added to baked goods or casseroles. By consuming 2 tablespoons of wheat bran, your stools will be softer and easier to pass. Remember when you increase bran intake; increase your water intake also.
- ✦ Try eating whole grain cereals and breads.
- ✦ Eat more vegetables, raw or cooked.
- ✦ Do light exercise after eating.
- ✦ Try drinking a hot beverage 30 minutes before the usual time for a bowel movement.

Shopping List for Constipation

- ✦ Barley
- ✦ Beans
- ✦ Bran
- ✦ Butter or margarine
- ✦ Canned broth
- ✦ Dijon mustard
- ✦ Eggs
- ✦ Fruit juices
- ✦ Ground sirloin

- ✦ Fruit, fresh, frozen, dried, canned
- ✦ Nuts
- ✦ Oatmeal
- ✦ Pasta
- ✦ Rice, wild, brown, white
- ✦ Prunes
- ✦ Raisins

- ✦ Seeds
- ✦ Spices and seasonings, dried or fresh
- ✦ Sugar cookie refrigerated slice and bake dough
- ✦ Sweet potatoes and potatoes

- ✦ Vegetables, fresh, frozen, canned
- ✦ Whipped topping, frozen
- ✦ Whole grain cereals and breads

Menus

Foods to eat to ease constipation.

Breakfast

94   Sweet Potato Pancakes with Apple Walnut Topping

124   Honey Bran Prune Muffins
    Egg of choice
    Orange Juice

201   Spinach Layered Dish
124   Banana Bran Muffins
    Fresh Fruit

Lunch

97   Mushroom Barley Soup
104   Chicken Salad
127   Oatmeal Chocolate Cake

102   Sweet Potato and Apple Soup
37   Tuna Salad
    Whole Wheat Toast

96   White Bean and Tortellini Soup

Salad Medley:

109   Black Bean and Corn Salad
103   Waldorf Salad
107   Tuna Pasta Salad
122   Zucchini Oatmeal-Raisin Muffins
93   Strawberry Raspberry Soup
116   Yam Veggie Wraps

Dinner

Comfort Food:

Meat Loaf   120
Basic Broccoli   111
Creamed Double Potatoes   141
Peach Crumble   128

One Dish Meals Suggestions:

Vegetable Lasagna   117
Southwestern Pasta   118
Chicken Tortilla Soup   206

Cream of Spinach Soup   205
Chicken with Bean Sauce   243
Baked Corn Casserole   111

Tropical Green Salad   232
Shrimp and Wild Rice Salad   106

Quick Veggie Soup   98
Italian Spinach Pie   194

Snacks

Avocado Soup   136

Granola   92

Strawberry Salsa   186

Cereal Mixture   181

Strawberry Slush   181

Couscous Salad   226

Granola

This crunchy mixture makes a great snack or just sprinkle it on fruit, yogurt or ice cream. Add whatever fruit combos you enjoy and throw in some nuts, if desired.

MAKES SIXTEEN (1/2-CUP) SERVINGS

4 cups old-fashioned oatmeal
1/2 cup wheat bran
2 tablespoons nonfat dry milk
1 teaspoon ground cinnamon
1/2 cup sunflower seeds
1/2 cup pumpkin seeds
2/3 cup honey
2 tablespoons molasses
1/2 cup dried cranberries
1 cup dried mixed fruit bits

Preheat oven to 300 degrees. Line a baking sheet with heavy foil to make clean up a snap. Mix together the oatmeal, bran, dry milk, cinnamon, sunflower and pumpkin seed and spread on the lined pan. In a small bowl, mix together the honey and molasses. Pour the honey mixture over the cereal, stirring and tossing until well coated. Place in the oven for 30 to 35 minutes, stirring every 15 minutes, and cooking until mixture is golden brown. Let cool and toss with the cranberries and dried mixed fruit.

Nutritional information per serving

Calories 228, Protein (g) 7, Carbohydrate (g) 39, Fat (g) 7, Cal. from Fat (%) 25, Saturated Fat (g) 1, Dietary Fiber (g) 4, Cholesterol (mg) 0, Sodium (mg) 10, Diabetic Exchanges: 1 starch, 0.5 fruit, 1 other carb., 1 fat

DOC'S NOTES:

Keep a jar of this for nibbles throughout the day. This beats the taste of any laxative. This is truly a great source of fiber. The fiber pulls fluid into the colon, softening the stool and aiding in bowel movements.

CONSTIPATION

Strawberry Raspberry Soup

A fabulous berry soup!

MAKES 12 SMALL SERVINGS

1 quart fresh strawberries, halved

3 cups fresh raspberries or 1 (12-ounce) package frozen raspberries, drained

1/2 cup plus 2/3 cup apple juice, divided

1/4 cup sugar

2 tablespoon cornstarch

1 cup water

1 tablespoon lemon juice

3/4 cup nonfat plain yogurt

1 1/2 teaspoons powdered sugar

1/2 teaspoon vanilla extract

Place the strawberries, raspberries, 1/2 cup apple juice, and sugar in a saucepan and let stand 15 minutes. Heat over low heat until boiling. Mix together the cornstarch and water, and stir into fruit mixture. Boil over low heat, stirring constantly, until fruits soften and soup is clear and thickened. Remove from heat and stir in the lemon juice. Chill. Before serving add remaining 2/3 cup apple juice to make soup consistency, or more if needed. In a small bowl, combine yogurt, powdered sugar, and vanilla. Serve soup in small bowls and top each with a tablespoon of yogurt mixture.

Nutritional information per serving

Calories 73, Protein (g) 2, Carbohydrate (g) 17, Fat (g) 0, Cal. from Fat (%) 0, Saturated Fat (g) 0, Dietary Fiber (g) 3, Cholesterol (mg) 0, Sodium (mg) 13, Diabetic Exchanges: 1 fruit

DOC'S NOTES:

High in Vitamin C and potassium as well as a good source of fiber.

Sweet Potato Pancakes with Apple Walnut Topping 🥕 ❄️

Use a shredding blade of the food processor for easy shredding. This incredible indulgent topping complements these pancakes and works great on ice cream.

MAKES ABOUT 18 PANCAKES

PANCAKES

6 cups shredded peeled sweet potatoes (yams)
1/4 cup all-purpose flour
1/2 teaspoon baking powder
1/8 teaspoon ground cinnamon
1 tablespoon honey
1 large egg
2 large egg whites
Apple Walnut Topping (recipe follows)

In a bowl, combine the shredded sweet potatoes, flour, baking powder, cinnamon, honey, egg, and egg whites with a fork until well blended. Heat a nonstick skillet coated with nonstick cooking spray, and drop about 2 tablespoons of batter (about 3 inches each) into hot pan. Flatten slightly with the spatula and cook pancakes over medium heat until golden on both sides. Set cooked pancakes on a plate and continue cooking until all batter is used. Serve with Apple Walnut Topping.

Note: Pancakes may be frozen or made ahead. To reheat, place on baking sheets and bake at 450 degrees for about 7 to 10 minutes or until crisp.

APPLE WALNUT TOPPING

1/2 cup light brown sugar
1/3 cup chopped walnuts
2 baking apples, peeled, core and thinly sliced
1 tablespoon orange juice
1/8 teaspoon ground cinnamon

In a skillet, add all the ingredients and cook over a medium-high heat, stirring, until the apples are tender and the brown sugar melts to form a syrup.

Nutritional information per serving
Calories 104, Protein (g) 2, Carbohydrate (g) 22, Fat (g) 2, Cal. from Fat (%) 15, Saturated Fat (g) 0, Dietary Fiber (g) 2, Cholesterol (mg) 12, Sodium (mg) 40, Diabetic Exchanges: 1 starch, 0.5 other carb.

DOC'S NOTES:

Sweet potatoes are high in beta carotene, fiber, and vitamins.

Tropical Salsa 🥕

This light tropical salsa is the perfect complement to any fish, pork, or chicken, or serve with chips.

MAKES 4 SERVINGS

1 (8-ounce) can pineapple chunks in its own juice, drained

1 tablespoon lemon juice

1/4 teaspoon ground ginger

1 1/2 tablespoons light brown sugar

1 (11-ounce) can mandarin orange segments, drained and coarsely chopped

2 green onions (scallions), chopped

1 teaspoon chopped pickled jalapeño peppers, optional

1 tablespoon cilantro, optional

In a medium bowl, coarsely chop the pineapple and add the lemon juice, ginger, brown sugar, coarsely chopped mandarin oranges, green onions, jalapeños, and cilantro; set aside. When ready to serve, heat, or serve at room temperature with your entrée.

Nutritional information per serving

Calories 74, Protein (g) 1, Carbohydrate (g) 19, Fat (g) 0, Cal. from Fat (%) 0, Saturated Fat (g) 0, Dietary Fiber (g) 1, Cholesterol (mg) 0, Sodium (mg) 28, Diabetic Exchanges: 1 fruit, 0.5 other carb.

DOC'S NOTES:

If the jalapeño peppers are too hot, just omit them. Great source of Vitamin C.

White Bean and Tortellini Soup 🥕 ❄️

For a quick, very tasty soup, try this recipe.

MAKES 8 SERVINGS

½ cup chopped green bell pepper
½ cup chopped celery
½ teaspoon minced garlic
8 cups canned fat-free chicken broth or
  vegetable broth
1 (6-ounce) package tri-colored tortellini
1 (15-ounce) can great Northern beans, drained
  and rinsed
1½ cups chopped tomatoes
1 teaspoon dried oregano leaves
1 teaspoon dried basil leaves
Salt and pepper to taste

In a large pot coated with nonstick cooking spray, sauté the green pepper, celery, and garlic until tender, about 5 to 7 minutes. Add chicken broth and bring to a boil. Add tortellini, reduce heat and cook 15 minutes or until tortellini is done. Add beans, tomatoes, oregano, basil, and salt and pepper. Continue cooking 5 minutes longer.

Nutritional information per serving
Calories 127, Protein (g) 9, Carbohydrate (g) 21,
Fat (g) 1, Cal. from Fat (%) 9, Saturated Fat (g) 1,
Dietary Fiber (g) 4, Cholesterol (mg) 11, Sodium (mg) 788,
Diabetic Exchanges: 0.5 very lean meat, 1 starch,
1 vegetable

DOC'S NOTES:

The beans are a great source of protein and fiber without any fat.

Mushroom Barley Soup 🥕 ❄️

A savory soup that hits the spot on a cool night. For a fast version, use quick cooking barley.

MAKES 8 SERVINGS

1 teaspoon minced garlic
1 onion, chopped
2 carrots, chopped
1/2 pound sliced mushrooms
1 cup shiitake mushrooms, sliced
1 (8-ounce) can tomato sauce
8 cups beef or vegetable broth
3/4 cup medium pearl barley
Salt and pepper to taste

In a large pot coated with nonstick cooking spray, sauté the garlic, onion, carrot, and mushrooms until tender. Add tomato sauce and broth. Bring to a boil and add barley. Reduce heat, cover, and cook for 1 hour or until barley is done. Season to taste. Add more water if needed.

Nutritional information per serving

Calories 118, Protein (g) 8, Carbohydrate (g) 21, Fat (g) 0, Cal. from Fat (%) 0, Saturated Fat (g) 0, Dietary Fiber (g) 4, Cholesterol (mg) 0, Sodium (mg) 1174, Diabetic Exchanges: 1 starch, 1.5 vegetable

DOC'S NOTES:

Soup and sandwich are quick and easy when you do not have a ravenous appetite. This provides fiber, B vitamins, copper, and beta carotene.

Quick Veggie Soup ✎ ❄

Any combination of cooked leftover vegetables may be substituted for the corn and carrots. Try adding some shredded cabbage to include a great cruciferous veggie.

MAKES 6 SERVINGS

1 onion, chopped
1 teaspoon minced garlic
1 (16-ounce) can tomato purée
4 cups water
Salt and pepper to taste
1 tablespoon Worcestershire sauce
1 small bay leaf
1 cup sliced carrots
1 (10-ounce) package frozen corn
1 (10-ounce) package frozen green peas
1/3 cup rice

In a large pot coated with nonstick cooking spray, sauté onions and garlic until softened, about 7 minutes. Add the tomato purée, water, salt and pepper, Worcestershire sauce, bay leaf, carrots, and corn. Bring to a boil and simmer for about 20 minutes. Add the peas and rice and simmer about 40 to 45 minutes longer or until the rice is done. Remove the bay leaf before serving. Add more water if needed while cooking to keep a soup consistency.

Nutritional information per serving

Calories 166, Protein (g) 7, Carbohydrate (g) 37, Fat (g) 1, Cal. from Fat (%) 4, Saturated Fat (g) 0, Dietary Fiber (g) 6, Cholesterol (mg) 0, Sodium (mg) 393, Diabetic Exchanges: 1.5 starch, 3 vegetable

DOC'S NOTES:

Freeze in small containers for those nights you just do not have the energy to cook. It provides Vitamin A, beta carotene, and fiber.

CONSTIPATION

Split Pea and Pasta Soup ❄

No need to take all day cooking split pea soup with this speedy updated recipe with old family flavor.

MAKES 5 TO 6 CUPS

1/2 cup chopped celery
1/2 cup chopped onion
2 (11 1/2-ounce) cans condensed split pea soup or any canned split pea soup
2 cups reduced sodium chicken broth
1 cup water
1 cup spaghetti, broken into 3 inch pieces, cooked and drained

In a pot coated with nonstick cooking spray, sauté the celery and onion until tender, about 5 minutes. Add the split pea soup, chicken broth and water. Cook until well heated and bubbly over medium heat. Add cooked pasta and serve.

Nutrition information per serving

Calories 228, Protein (g) 12, Carbohydrate (g) 38, Fat (g) 3, Calories from Fat (%) 13, Saturated Fat (g) 2, Dietary Fiber (g) 5, Cholesterol (mg) 4, Sodium (mg) 847, Diabetic Exchanges: 1 very lean meat, 2.5 starch

Squash Bisque

You may substitute two (10-ounce) packages frozen squash for fresh. This delicious soup will attract squash fans.

MAKES EIGHT (1-CUP) SERVINGS

2 tablespoons olive oil

1 medium onion, chopped

1¼ pounds yellow squash, thinly sliced

1 cup diced carrots, about 2

2 large Yukon potatoes, peeled and diced

4 cups canned fat-free chicken broth or vegetable broth

¼ teaspoon dried thyme leaves

Dash of paprika

Salt and pepper to taste

In a large pot, heat oil and sauté onion until tender, about 5 minutes. Add the squash and sauté, stirring, about 10 minutes. Add carrots, potato and chicken broth. Bring to a boil. Reduce heat and simmer about 30 to 40 minutes or until veggies are tender. Add thyme, paprika, and salt and pepper to taste.

Nutritional information per serving

Calories 97, Protein (g) 4, Carbohydrate (g) 15, Fat (g) 4, Cal. from Fat (%) 30, Saturated Fat (g) 1, Dietary Fiber (g) 3, Cholesterol (mg) 0, Sodium (mg) 317, Diabetic Exchanges: 0.5 starch, 1.5 vegetable, 1 fat

DOC'S NOTES:

Squash is packed with nutrients and is an excellent source of Vitamin C and potassium.

Minestrone

A variety of vegetables and white beans with Italian flair

MAKES 10 CUPS

1 onion, chopped

½ cup chopped celery

1 teaspoon minced garlic

2 (14½-ounce) cans diced tomatoes with juice

3 (14-ounce) cans vegetable broth or
chicken broth

1 bay leaf

1 tablespoon dried oregano leaves

1 teaspoon dried basil leaves

1 red potato, peeled and diced

1 cup coarsely chopped carrots

½ pound mushrooms, thinly sliced

2 cups zucchini, halved lengthwise and
thinly sliced

1/3 cup dry elbow macaroni

1 (16-ounce) cannelloni or white beans, drained
and rinsed

1½ cups fresh baby spinach leaves

Salt and pepper to taste

In a large pot coated with nonstick cooking spray, sauté the onion, celery and garlic until tender. Add diced tomatoes, vegetable broth, bay leaf, oregano, basil, potato, carrots, mushrooms and zucchini. Bring to a boil, reduce heat, and cover, simmering for 15 minutes. Add the pasta and continue cooking for another 15 minutes or until the pasta is done and the vegetables are tender. Stir in the beans and spinach, cooking until well heated. Season to taste and remove bay leaf.

Nutrition information per serving
Calories 103, Protein (g) 5, Carbohydrate (g) 21,
Fat (g) 0, Calories from Fat (%) 0, Saturated Fat (g) 0,
Dietary Fiber (g) 4, Cholesterol (mg) 0, Sodium (mg) 906,
Diabetic Exchanges: 1 starch, 1.5 vegetable

CONSTIPATION

Sweet Potato and Apple Soup

By blending sweet potatoes and apples with a touch of ginger and curry, you have an incredibly flavored soup that leaves a lasting impression. The toasty walnuts add the finishing touch to make this a perfect fall soup. Make ahead and refrigerate. If reheating, add more milk as needed to reach soup consistency.

MAKES FIVE (1-CUP) SERVINGS

1/2 cup chopped onions
4 cups peeled and chopped sweet potatoes (yams)
2 cups peeled, cored, and chopped baking apples
2 cups canned fat-free chicken broth
1/2 teaspoon ground ginger
1/2 teaspoon ground curry
1 tablespoon honey
1 cup skim milk
1/3 cup chopped walnuts, toasted

In a nonstick pot coated with nonstick cooking spray, sauté the onions until tender. Add the sweet potatoes, apples, chicken broth, ginger, curry, and honey. Bring to a boil. Reduce heat, cover, and simmer until the potatoes are tender, about 25 minutes. Transfer to a food processor and purée until smooth. Return to pot; stir in the milk until blended. Sprinkle each serving with toasted walnuts.

Nutritional information per serving

Calories 233, Protein (g) 6, Carbohydrate (g) 41, Fat (g) 6, Cal. from Fat (%) 22, Saturated Fat (g) 1, Dietary Fiber (g) 5, Cholesterol (mg) 1, Sodium (mg) 288, Diabetic Exchanges: 2 starch, 0.5 fruit, 1 fat

DOC'S NOTES:

Sweet potatoes and apples are a great source of fiber and nutrition.

Waldorf Salad

This recipe is a healthy update on a classic. The salad is an excellent source of fiber, vitamins and minerals.

MAKES **8** TO **10** SERVINGS

6 cups chopped apples (red and green)
2 stalks celery, chopped
1 cup red or green seedless grapes
1/2 cup chopped walnuts, toasted
1/2 cup raisins
1 cup nonfat plain yogurt
1/4 cup light mayonnaise
1/4 cup fresh orange juice

In a mixing bowl combine apples, celery, grapes, walnuts, and raisins. In another bowl, mix yogurt, mayonnaise, and orange juice. Toss the dressing with the salad ingredients and chill.

Nutritional information per serving
Calories 153, Protein (g) 3, Carbohydrate (g) 24, Fat (g) 6, Cal. from Fat (%) 35, Saturated Fat (g) 1, Dietary Fiber (g) 3, Cholesterol (mg) 3, Sodium (mg) 76, Diabetic Exchanges: 1.5 fruit, 1 fat

DOC'S NOTES:

This is not only filled with fiber, but is very colorful and will surely stimulate your taste buds. For added calories, don't use fat-free products.

Chicken Salad

Use leftover chicken to create this delicious salad filled with fruit and flavor.

MAKES 6 TO 8 SERVINGS

3 cups cooked chicken breasts, cut in chunks.
1 cup chopped celery
3/4 pound red and green grapes
1/3 cup light mayonnaise
1 tablespoon lemon juice
1 tablespoon soy sauce
1 large apple, chopped
1/4 cup pecans, toasted

In a large bowl, combine chicken, celery, and grapes. In a small bowl, mix together mayonnaise, lemon juice, and soy sauce. Toss dressing with chicken mixture. Refrigerate until serving. Just before serving, mix in apples and pecans.

Nutritional information per serving

Calories 193, Protein (g) 17, Carbohydrate (g) 14, Fat (g) 8, Cal. from Fat (%) 37, Saturated Fat (g) 1, Dietary Fiber (g) 2, Cholesterol (mg) 48, Sodium (mg) 241, Diabetic Exchanges: 2 very lean meat, 1 fruit, 1 fat

DOC'S NOTES:

You will find this salad to be a great source of fiber. Great dish to enjoy if your bowels are a bit sluggish. Apples are a great source of fiber.

CONSTIPATION

Mandarin Chicken Salad

This super chicken salad combined with fruit and water chestnut; and tossed with a light lemon dressing is hard to beat.

MAKES 4 TO 6 SERVINGS

1½ pounds skinless, boneless chicken breasts, cut into chunks

1 tablespoon canola oil

4 tablespoons reduced-sodium soy sauce, divided

½ teaspoon minced garlic

¼ teaspoon ground ginger

1 cup green grapes, cut in half

1 cup chopped celery

½ cup chopped green onions (scallions)

1 (11-ounce) can mandarin orange segments in water, drained

1 (8-ounce) can sliced water chestnuts, drained

1 (6-ounce) container nonfat lemon yogurt

6 cups (loosely packed) washed, stemmed, torn spinach leaves

In a bowl, combine the chicken, oil, 2 tablespoons soy sauce, garlic, and ginger, coating the chicken well. In a skillet coated with nonstick cooking spray, cook the chicken mixture over medium heat, about 5 to 7 minutes, until the chicken is done. Set aside and let cool. In a bowl, combine the chicken, grapes, celery, green onions, orange segments, and water chestnuts. Mix together the yogurt and remaining 2 tablespoons soy sauce and pour over the chicken mixture. Cover and refrigerate until the mixture is well chilled, about 2 hours. Serve on the spinach leaves.

Nutritional information per serving

Calories 241, Protein (g) 30, Carbohydrate (g) 21, Fat (g) 4, Cal. from Fat (%) 15, Saturated Fat (g) 1, Dietary Fiber (g) 3, Cholesterol (mg) 66, Sodium (mg) 542, Diabetic Exchanges: 3 very lean meat, 1 fruit, 1 vegetable

DOC'S NOTES:

This is filled with fiber and Vitamin C. This is a great salad to help keep those bowels moving.

Shrimp and Wild Rice Salad

Adjust the veggies in this salad to your preference and availability. For a vegetarian delight, just delete the shrimp.

MAKES 6 SERVINGS

1 (6-ounce) box long-grain and wild rice
1 cup cooked rice
4 cups broccoli florets
1 pound cooked and peeled medium shrimp
1 cup sliced carrots
1/2 pound mushrooms, sliced
1 cup thinly sliced zucchini
1 cup thinly sliced yellow squash
1/2 cup red bell pepper, cored and chopped
1 bunch green onions (scallions), chopped
3 large hard-boiled eggs, whites only,
   finely chopped
2/3 cup nonfat plain yogurt
3 tablespoons light mayonnaise
Salt and pepper to taste

Cook the wild rice according to package directions; set aside. In a large bowl, combine the wild rice, rice, broccoli, shrimp, carrots, mushrooms, zucchini, squash, red pepper, onions, and egg whites. In a small bowl, stir together the yogurt and mayonnaise. Pour the yogurt mixture over the shrimp mixture; toss lightly. Season with salt and pepper. Cover and refrigerate.

Nutritional information per serving

Calories 306, Protein (g) 26, Carbohydrate (g) 42, Fat (g) 4, Cal. from Fat (%) 12, Saturated Fat (g) 1, Dietary Fiber (g) 4, Cholesterol (mg) 151, Sodium (mg) 724, Diabetic Exchanges: 3 very lean meat, 2 starch, 2 vegetable

DOC'S NOTES:

A cup of this salad makes a great snack any time of day. It is high in fiber and contains beta carotene, vitamins, minerals, and a cruciferous vegetable.

Tuna Pasta Salad

This simple and sensational salad takes tuna to a new level.

MAKES 6 TO 8 SERVINGS

1 (16-ounce) package tri-colored rotini
1 bunch fresh broccoli cut into florets
2 medium tomatoes, cut into chunks
1/4 cup pitted ripe olives, chopped
1/2 onion, cut into thin slices, rings separated
1 (12-ounce) can solid white tuna in spring
  water, drained
1/3 cup balsamic vinegar
1/4 cup lemon juice
1 tablespoon water
2 tablespoons olive oil
2 tablespoons Dijon mustard
1/2 teaspoon pepper

Cook the pasta according to package directions, omitting any salt and oil. Drain and combine with the broccoli florets, tomatoes, olives, onion, and tuna. Set aside. In a small bowl, combine the vinegar, lemon juice, water, olive oil, mustard, and pepper. Beat with a fork vigorously. Pour over the pasta mixture. Toss gently. Chill 2 hours. Toss gently before serving.

Nutritional information per serving

Calories 336, Protein (g) 19, Carbohydrate (g) 50,
Fat (g) 6, Cal. from Fat (%) 17, Saturated Fat (g) 1,
Dietary Fiber (g) 3, Cholesterol (mg) 18, Sodium (mg) 292,
Diabetic Exchanges: 1.5 very lean meat, 3 starch,
1 vegetable

DOC'S NOTES:

Good source of protein and fiber as well as Vitamins A and C. Broccoli provides your cruciferous vegetable which is linked to cancer protection.

Black and White Bean Salad

Here's an updated bean salad with a Southwestern flair. Add beans of your choice.

MAKES EIGHT (1/2-CUP) SERVINGS

1 (15-ounce) can white (cannellini or navy) beans, rinsed and drained
1 (15-ounce) can black beans, rinsed and drained
1 cup chopped tomato
1 cup chopped green onions (scallions)
1/2 cup chopped red bell pepper
1/2 cup picante sauce
1/4 cup balsamic vinegar
1/2 teaspoon minced garlic
1 tablespoon olive oil
2 tablespoons chopped fresh cilantro, optional

In a large bowl, combine white beans, black beans, tomato, green onions, and red pepper. In a small bowl, whisk together picante sauce, balsamic vinegar, garlic, olive oil, and cilantro. Toss with salad and refrigerate until serving.

Nutritional information per serving
Calories 125, Protein (g) 5, Carbohydrate (g) 20, Fat (g) 2, Cal. from Fat (%) 18, Saturated Fat (g) 0, Dietary Fiber (g) 6, Cholesterol (mg) 0, Sodium (mg) 364, Diabetic Exchanges: 1 starch, 1 vegetable

DOC'S NOTES:

Beans are high in protein, carbs, and fiber.

Black Bean and Corn Salad

A quick and delicious salad that adds to any plate. Serve with chicken or fish as a condiment.

MAKES 6 SERVINGS

1 (15-ounce) can black beans, drained and rinsed
1 (11-ounce) can golden sweet corn, drained
1 tomato, chopped
1/4 cup fresh chopped cilantro
2 tablespoons chopped red onion
3 tablespoons lemon juice
2 tablespoons olive oil
Salt and pepper to taste

Combine all ingredients in bowl. Refrigerate until ready to serve.

Nutritional information per serving

Calories 142, Protein (g) 5, Carbohydrate (g) 19, Fat (g) 6, Cal. from Fat (%) 34, Saturated Fat (g) 1, Dietary Fiber (g) 5, Cholesterol (mg) 0, Sodium (mg) 294, Diabetic Exchanges: 0.5 very lean meat, 1.5 starch, 1 fat

Baked Beans ✎ ❄

This is an easy version of an old-fashioned recipe. If desired, you can leave out the bacon for a vegetarian dish.

MAKES 12 SERVINGS

1 onion, chopped
1 green bell pepper, cored and chopped
3 ounces Canadian bacon,
   cut in 1/2-inch pieces, optional
2 (15-ounce) cans red kidney beans, drained
2 (19-ounce) cans white kidney beans
   (cannellini), drained
2 tablespoons Worcestershire sauce
1/3 cup light brown sugar
2/3 cup barbecue sauce
1 teaspoon dry mustard

Preheat oven to 350 degrees. In a large skillet coated with nonstick cooking spray, sauté the onion and green pepper until tender, about 4 minutes. Add the Canadian bacon. Cook for 5 minutes longer. Place all the beans in a 2-quart casserole dish and add the sautéed vegetables, Worcestershire sauce, brown sugar, barbecue sauce, and mustard. Mix well. Bake, covered, for 40 minutes.

Nutritional information per serving
Calories 184, Protein (g) 8, Carbohydrate (g) 34, Fat (g) 1, Cal. from Fat (%) 6, Saturated Fat (g) 0, Dietary Fiber (g) 8, Cholesterol (mg) 0, Sodium (mg) 472, Diabetic Exchanges: 0.5 very lean meat, 2 starch, 1 vegetable

DOC'S NOTES:

Beans provide a good source of protein, potassium, and iron.

Basic Broccoli 🥕

Broccoli with flavor. For a time saver, buy broccoli crowns.

MAKES 4 TO 6 SERVINGS

4 to 6 cups broccoli florets
1/2 cup water
1/2 teaspoon chicken bouillon granules
  (or 1/2 cup chicken broth but delete water)

In microwave-safe dish, place all ingredients. Cover with plastic wrap and microwave for 6 to 8 minutes or until broccoli is tender.

Nutritional information per serving
Calories 22, Protein (g) 2, Carbohydrate (g) 4,
Fat (g) 0, Cal. from Fat (%) 0, Saturated Fat (g) 0,
Dietary Fiber (g) 2, Cholesterol (mg) 0, Sodium (mg) 159,
Diabetic Exchanges: 1 vegetable

DOC'S NOTES:

Broccoli is a cruciferous family veggie. The indoles found in broccoli are felt to be effective In protecting against certain forms of cancer.

Baked Corn Casserole 🥕 ❄

Use plain canned tomatoes for a less spicy version.

MAKES 6 SERVINGS

1 cup onion, chopped
1 tablespoon margarine
1 (10-ounce) can diced tomatoes and green chiles
1 (16-ounce) can whole-kernel yellow corn, drained
1 (15-ounce) can shoe peg white corn, drained
1 (15-ounce) can cream-style corn

In a pot, sauté onion in margarine until soft. Add tomatoes, whole-kernel corn, shoe peg corn, and creamed corn. Refrigerate for at least 8 hours or overnight. Bake at 325 degrees for 1 hour.

Nutritional information per serving
Calories 191, Protein (g) 5, Carbohydrate (g) 39,
Fat (g) 3, Cal. from Fat (%) 14, Saturated Fat (g) 1,
Dietary Fiber (g) 4, Cholesterol (mg) 0, Sodium (mg) 700,
Diabetic Exchanges: 2.5 starch, 1 vegetable

DOC'S NOTES:

Tomatoes provide Vitamins A and C.

Tasty Brown Rice

Here's a little twist to jazz up your rice. Brown rice adds flavor and fiber. The veggies may be omitted for a basic brown rice recipe.

MAKES 6 TO 8 SERVINGS

1 tablespoon olive oil
1/2 cup finely chopped onion
1/2 teaspoon minced garlic
1 (16-ounce) package assorted veggies (broccoli, carrot, and snow peas), about 8 cups
1 cup brown rice
1/2 cup diced tomato
1 bay leaf
1 3/4 cups canned fat-free chicken broth
1/2 cup water
3 tablespoons grated Parmesan cheese

In a large pot, heat olive oil and sauté the onion, garlic and assorted veggies over medium heat, stirring until tender. Add the rice, tomato, bay leaf, broth and water. Stir until well mixed. Cover and bring to a boil. Reduce heat and cook until rice is done, about 20 to 30 minutes. Remove bay leaf. Stir in cheese.

Nutritional information per serving

Calories 141, Protein (g) 5, Carbohydrate (g) 23, Fat (g) 3, Cal. from Fat (%) 20, Saturated Fat (g) 1, Dietary Fiber (g) 2, Cholesterol (mg) 2, Sodium (mg) 199, Diabetic Exchanges: 1 starch, 0.5 fat, 1 vegetable

DOC'S NOTES:

The brown rice is the only rice that contains vitamin E. The vegetables are a great source of fiber.

CONSTIPATION

Wild Rice and Barley Pilaf 🥕

A nice alternative to replace a rice dish.

MAKES 6 TO 8 SERVINGS

1 (6-ounce) package long grain and wild rice
1/2 cup pearl barley
3 cups canned fat-free chicken broth or
    vegetable broth
1 tablespoon margarine
1/3 cup sliced almonds, toasted

Preheat oven to 325 degrees. In saucepan, combine rice, seasoning packet, barley, chicken broth, and margarine. Bring to a boil. Reduce heat, cover, and simmer for 10 minutes. Spoon into a 1½-quart casserole dish. Bake, covered, for 1 hour or until rice and barley are tender and liquid is absorbed. Fluff rice mixture with a fork; stir in almonds.

Nutritional information per serving

Calories 162, Protein (g) 5, Carbohydrate (g) 28, Fat (g) 4, Cal. from Fat (%) 20, Saturated Fat (g) 0, Dietary Fiber (g) 3, Cholesterol (mg) 0, Sodium (mg) 566, Diabetic Exchanges: 2 starch, 0.5 fat

DOC'S NOTES:

Rice, salad and a grilled chicken breast is quick, simple, and filling. The wild rice and barley provide a good source of fiber.

Veggie Angel Hair 🥕

You can substitute your favorite veggies to create a version that suits your taste buds. This is a great veggie dish or main dish on a meatless night.

MAKES 4 MAIN DISH SERVINGS,
   6 TO 8 SIDE SERVINGS

1 (16-ounce) package angel hair pasta
2 tablespoons olive oil
1 cup chopped onion
1 tablespoon minced garlic
2 medium zucchini, cut into 2×1/2-inch pieces
1 cup frozen corn
1/4 cup water
1 teaspoon dried dill weed leaves
1/4 cup grated Parmesan cheese
1/4 cup chopped pecans, toasted, optional

Cook the pasta according to package directions until done. Drain and set aside. In a large skillet heat the olive oil, sauté the onion and garlic until tender. Add the zucchini, corn and 1/4 cup water to the skillet, cover and cook the vegetables over medium heat about 5 minutes, or until just tender. Add the pasta and toss with dill and Parmesan cheese, stirring until heated through. Mix in pecans, if desired.

Nutritional information per main dish serving
Calories 469, Protein (g) 16, Carbohydrate (g) 79, Fat (g) 11, Cal. from Fat (%) 20, Saturated Fat (g) 2, Dietary Fiber (g) 5, Cholesterol (mg) 5, Sodium (mg) 129, Diabetic Exchanges: 5 starch, 1 vegetable, 1 fat

DOC'S NOTES:

The skin of the squash is a great source of beta-carotene.

CONSTIPATION

Creamy Squash Casserole 🥕

Here's another way to turn squash into an incredible dish. Make ahead and refrigerate; pop into a cold oven to bake.

MAKES 6 TO 8 SERVINGS

2 pounds yellow squash (about 8), sliced
1 cup nonfat plain yogurt
Salt and pepper to taste
1/2 teaspoon dried basil leaves
1/2 cup dry bread crumbs
1/4 cup shredded reduced-fat sharp Cheddar cheese, optional
1 tablespoon margarine, melted
1/2 teaspoon paprika

Preheat oven to 350 degrees. Coat a 1 1/2-quart casserole dish with nonstick cooking spray. Boil the squash in a saucepan in a small amount of water over a medium to high heat until tender, about 5 minutes. Drain well. Combine the squash with yogurt, salt and pepper, and basil in a mixing bowl. Pour into the casserole dish. Combine the bread crumbs, Cheddar cheese, margarine, and paprika. Sprinkle over the squash mixture. Bake for 20 minutes.

Nutritional information per serving

Calories 84, Protein (g) 4, Carbohydrate (g) 13, Fat (g) 2, Cal. from Fat (%) 22, Saturated Fat (g) 0, Dietary Fiber (g) 3, Cholesterol (mg) 1, Sodium (mg) 101, Diabetic Exchanges: 0.5 starch, 1 vegetable

DOC'S NOTES:

Squash is low in fiber so here's a great way to include a veggie at this time.

Yam Veggie Wraps

A quick and wonderful flavor combo that makes a nutritious wrap to remember. Shred sweet potatoes on grater or in a food processor.

MAKES 6 WRAPS

1 sweet potato (yam), peeled and shredded
(about 1 cup)
½ cup chopped red onion
1 cup black beans, rinsed and drained
2 green onions (scallions), chopped
¼ cup sunflower seeds
2 tablespoons light Italian or Caesar dressing
1 teaspoon honey
6 flour tortillas, warmed to soften

In a skillet coated with nonstick cooking spray, sauté shredded yams over medium high heat for about 5 minutes or until crisp tender. Transfer to a bowl. In same skillet coated with nonstick cooking spray, sauté red onion for about 5 minutes until tender. Add sautéed onion, black beans, green onions, and sunflower seeds to shredded yams, mixing well. In a small bowl, mix together dressing and honey and toss with yam mixture to coat. Fill tortillas with mixture and wrap.

Nutritional information per serving
Calories 200, Protein (g) 7, Carbohydrate (g) 32, Fat (g) 5, Cal. from Fat (%) 23, Saturated Fat (g) 1, Dietary Fiber (g) 5, Cholesterol (mg) 0, Sodium (mg) 231, Diabetic Exchanges: 2 starch, 0.5 fat

DOC'S NOTES:

Sweet Potatoes are one of the most nutritious vegetables.

Vegetable Lasagna ✏️ ❄️

Lasagna makes a great meal, freezes well, and can be made ahead.

MAKES 12 SERVINGS

1 onion, chopped
3 cloves garlic, minced
1 green bell pepper, cored and chopped
1 (6-ounce) can tomato paste
1 (10-ounce) can diced tomatoes and green chiles
1 (10-ounce) can stewed tomatoes
1 (11 1/2-ounce) can tomato juice
1 teaspoon dried basil leaves
1 teaspoon dried oregano leaves
1 teaspoon dried thyme leaves
1 1/2 tablespoons red wine vinegar
1 bay leaf
1/2 pound fresh mushrooms, sliced
1/2 cup shredded carrot
1 bunch broccoli flowerets
1/2 pound lasagna noodles
1 1/2 cups shredded part-skim mozzarella cheese

Preheat oven to 350 degrees. Coat a large skillet with nonstick cooking spray and add onion, garlic and green pepper. Sauté until tender. Add tomato paste, diced tomatoes and green chiles, stewed tomatoes, and tomato juice. Bring to a boil. Add remaining ingredients except lasagna noodles and cheese. Reduce heat and simmer at least 30 minutes or until vegetables are tender and sauce has slightly thickened. Discard bay leaf. Cook lasagna noodles according to directions on package omitting salt and oil; drain. Spoon some vegetable sauce over the bottom of a 3-quart oblong baking dish. Layer one-third each of lasagna noodles, Cheese Mixture (recipe follows), remaining vegetable sauce, and mozzarella cheese. Repeat layers twice. Bake, covered, for 30 minutes. Let stand 10 minutes before cutting.

CHEESE MIXTURE

2 cups low fat cottage cheese
1 large egg white
2 tablespoons chopped parsley
1/4 cup grated Parmesan cheese

Combine all ingredients in a food processor, blending well.

Nutritional information per serving

Calories 192, Protein (g) 14, Carbohydrate (g) 26, Fat (g) 4, Cal. from Fat (%) 17, Saturated Fat (g) 2, Dietary Fiber (g) 3, Cholesterol (mg) 12, Sodium (mg) 558, Diabetic Exchanges: 1.5 lean meat, 1 starch, 2 vegetable

DOC'S NOTES:

Filled with Vitamins A, C, and minerals. Broccoli provides the cruciferous vegetable.

Southwestern Pasta

Vegetarians as well as pasta lovers will put this southwestern recipe high on their lists. Place tomatoes in food processor to purée or purchase diced tomatoes.

MAKES 6 TO 8 SERVINGS

1 (28-ounce) can no-salt added whole tomatoes, puréed, with their juice

1 onion, chopped

1½ teaspoons chili powder

½ teaspoon ground cumin

1 teaspoon dried oregano leaves

½ teaspoon minced garlic

¼ teaspoon ground cinnamon

¼ teaspoon red pepper flakes, optional

Salt and pepper to taste

1 (16-ounce) package rotini

1 (16-ounce) can black beans, drained and rinsed

1 (10-ounce) package frozen corn

1 (4½-ounce) can chopped green chiles, drained

1 cup shredded reduced-fat Cheddar cheese, optional

Heat a large pot coated with nonstick cooking spray to medium heat, and add the tomato purée, onion, chili powder, cumin, oregano, garlic, sugar, cinnamon, red pepper flakes, and salt and pepper. Bring to a boil, reduce heat, and simmer, covered, to blend the flavors, 20 to 25 minutes. Meanwhile, cook the pasta according to package directions, omitting any oil and salt. Drain well. Stir the black beans, corn, and green chiles into the sauce. Cook until the corn is crisp-tender, about 5 minutes. Remove from the heat. To serve, toss the black bean mixture with the pasta. If desired, serve with reduced-fat Cheddar cheese.

Nutritional information per serving

Calories 321, Protein (g) 13, Carbohydrate (g) 64, Fat (g) 2, Cal. from Fat (%) 5, Saturated Fat (g) 0, Dietary Fiber (g) 8, Cholesterol (mg) 0, Sodium (mg) 254, Diabetic Exchanges: 4 starch, 1 vegetable

DOC'S NOTES:

The tomatoes are a good source of vitamins A, C, E and lycopene while the beans, corn and chiles are a good source of fiber.

CONSTIPATION

Shrimp and Squash Scampi ❄

Shrimp and squash pair to make a superb meal.

MAKES 4 SERVINGS

1 (8-ounce) package small pasta or orzo
2 tablespoons olive oil
1 pound zucchini, halved lengthwise and sliced
1 pound yellow squash, halved lengthwise and sliced
1 pound medium shrimp, peeled
1 tablespoon minced garlic
3/4 cup clam juice or chicken broth
2 tablespoons lemon juice
2 tablespoons chopped parsley
1/4 cup grated Parmesan cheese, optional

Cook the pasta according to package directions. Drain; set aside. Meanwhile, in a large skillet, heat the olive oil over a medium high heat and stir fry the zucchini and squash until crisp tender, about 5 minutes. Add the shrimp and continue cooking for another 5 minutes or until the shrimp are almost done. Add the garlic, clam juice, and lemon juice, cooking until the shrimp are done, about 3 to 5 minutes. Add the parsley, pasta, and Parmesan cheese, tossing to mix well.

Nutritional information per serving

Calories 412, Protein (g) 27, Carbohydrate (g) 52, Fat (g) 11, Cal. from Fat (%) 23, Saturated Fat (g) 3, Dietary Fiber (g) 5, Cholesterol (mg) 140, Sodium (mg) 582, Diabetic Exchanges: 2 very lean meat, 3 starch, 2 vegetable, 1 fat

CONSTIPATION

Meat Loaf ✳

Sometimes a comfort food such as meat loaf hits the spot. The chili sauce topping adds that finishing touch. Raid a salad bar for shredded carrots. Cut recipe in half and place in smaller loaf pan for smaller meat loaf.

MAKES 6 TO 8 SERVINGS

1½ pounds ground sirloin
2 large egg whites
1 carrot, shredded (about ½ cup)
1 teaspoon dried oregano leaves
1 teaspoon dried basil leaves
Salt and pepper to taste
½ cup old-fashioned oatmeal
1 cup tomato juice
⅓ cup chili sauce

Preheat oven to 350 degrees. Mix together ground sirloin, egg whites, carrot, oregano, basil, and salt and pepper. In a small bowl, mix together oatmeal and tomato juice, let sit for 5 minutes and combine with meat mixture. Transfer to a 9×5×3-inch loaf pan and bake for 40 minutes. Remove from oven and cover top with chili sauce. Return to oven for 20 minutes longer. Drain any excess grease.

Nutritional information per serving
Calories 188, Protein (g) 20, Carbohydrate (g) 9, Fat (g) 8, Cal. from Fat (%) 39, Saturated Fat (g) 3, Dietary Fiber (g) 1, Cholesterol (mg) 31, Sodium (mg) 340, Diabetic Exchanges: 2.5 lean meat, 0.5 starch

DOC'S NOTES:

The meat is a good source of protein and ground sirloin is a very lean cut of meat.

CONSTIPATION

All Natural Laxative 🥕

This is not a flavor savor but it works.

MAKES 18 (2 TABLESPOON) SERVINGS

1¼ cups unprocessed bran
1 cup prune juice
1 tablespoon molasses or honey
1 cup applesauce

Mix and store in a covered container in the refrigerator for up to 7 days. Stir before taking. Take 2 tablespoons every night as needed.

Nutritional information per serving

Calories 28, Protein (g) 1, Carbohydrate (g) 7, Fat (g) 0, Cal. from Fat (%) 0, Saturated Fat (g) 0, Dietary Fiber (g) 2, Cholesterol (mg) 0, Sodium (mg) 1, Diabetic Exchanges: 0.5 fruit

DOC'S NOTES:

If 2 tablespoons caused diarrhea, decrease to 1 tablespoon. If you find that 2 tablespoons is not enough, you can increase to 3 or 4 tablespoons. If this combination is not working, you can also take a laxative. The prune juice comes in 6 packs of (5½-ounce) cans. The high fiber content acts by drawing water into the colon, softening your stool and aiding in bowel movements. Always drink fluids to increase the effectiveness of the fiber.

Zucchini Oatmeal-
Raisin Muffins

These are a grainy not so sweet muffin. Their versatility makes them great for breakfast, a snack, or with a bowl of soup or salad.

MAKES 12 MUFFINS

1 1/2 cups buttermilk

1 cup old-fashioned oatmeal

2 tablespoons margarine, softened

1/2 cup light brown sugar

1 large egg, lightly beaten

1/2 cup all-purpose flour

1 cup whole wheat flour

1 teaspoon baking powder

1 teaspoon baking soda

1 teaspoon ground cinnamon

1 cup shredded zucchini

1/2 cup golden raisins

Preheat oven to 400 degrees. In a medium bowl, stir together the buttermilk and oatmeal; set aside for 15 minutes. In another mixing bowl, cream together the margarine and brown sugar. Beat in the egg. In another bowl, combine the flours, baking powder, baking soda, and cinnamon. Add the oatmeal mixture alternately with the dry ingredients to the creamed mixture and stir to combine. Stir in the zucchini and raisins.

Divide the batter among the muffin tin cups and bake for 20 to 25 minutes, or until a toothpick inserted in the center of a muffin comes out clean.

Nutritional information per serving
Calories 170, Protein (g) 5, Carbohydrate (g) 32, Fat (g) 3, Cal. from Fat (%) 17, Saturated Fat (g) 1, Dietary Fiber (g) 3, Cholesterol (mg) 19, Sodium (mg) 211, Diabetic Exchanges: 1 starch, 0.5 fruit, 0.5 other carb., 0.5 fat

DOC'S NOTES:

I recommend a high fiber muffin such as this one daily. If you are taking any type narcotic pain medicine, you need the extra fiber daily. The narcotic medicines slow the normal contractile activity of the bowels, leading to constipation. By adding fiber and fluids, you promote bowel activity.

Sweet Potato, Apple, and Walnut Muffins

The tartness of apples and raisins combined with the sweetness of yams and flavorful walnuts create a moist muffin that will quickly become one of your favorites.

MAKES 18 MUFFINS

1³/4 cups all-purpose flour
1¹/2 teaspoons baking powder
1 teaspoon ground cinnamon
3 tablespoons canola oil
³/4 cup light brown sugar
1 large egg
1 large egg white
1 (15-ounce) can sweet potatoes (yams),
  drained and mashed
¹/2 cup skim milk
1³/4 cups chopped and peeled baking apples
¹/3 cup chopped walnuts
¹/3 cup golden raisins

Preheat oven to 400 degrees. Coat 18 muffin tin cups with nonstick cooking spray or line with paper liners. In a bowl, mix together flour, baking powder, and cinnamon; set aside.

In another bowl, mix together the oil, brown sugar, egg, egg white, mashed sweet potatoes, and milk until well mixed. Make a well in the center of the dry ingredients and add potato mixture, stirring until moistened. Do not overmix. Fold in the apples, walnuts, and raisins. Spoon batter into prepared muffin tins, filling about three-fourths full. Bake for 20 to 25 minutes or until done.

Nutritional information per serving

Calories 150, Protein (g) 3, Carbohydrate (g) 26, Fat (g) 4, Cal. from Fat (%) 25, Saturated Fat (g) 0, Dietary Fiber (g) 1, Cholesterol (mg) 12, Sodium (mg) 62, Diabetic Exchanges: 1 starch, 0.5 fruit, 0.5 other carb., 0.5 fat

DOC'S NOTES:

Apples provide fiber, Vitamin C, potassium and boron. Apples are fibrous, juicy, and non-sticky, making them a good tooth cleaner and gum stimulator.

Honey Bran Prune Muffins 🥕 ❄️

High fiber in a tasty muffin.

MAKES 18 MUFFINS

2 cups wheat bran
2 cups all-purpose flour
1/8 teaspoon salt
1 teaspoon baking soda
1/2 cup light brown sugar
3 large eggs
1 cup prune juice
1/2 cup canola oil or applesauce
1/2 cup honey
1 cup raisins

Preheat oven to 400 degrees. In a bowl, combine bran, flour, salt, baking soda, and brown sugar. Add eggs, prune juice, oil or applesauce, and honey, mixing well. Stir in raisins. Pour batter into paper lined muffin tins. Bake for 20 minutes.

Nutritional information per serving

Calories 219, Protein (g) 4, Carbohydrate (g) 38, Fat (g) 7, Cal. from Fat (%) 28, Saturated Fat (g) 1, Dietary Fiber (g) 4, Cholesterol (mg) 35, Sodium (mg) 103, Diabetic Exchanges: 1 starch, 1 other carb., 0.5 fruit, 1 fat

Banana Bran Muffins 🥕 ❄️

Yummy! Wheat bran is found in the health food section in grocery stores.

MAKES 12 MUFFINS

1 cup all-purpose flour
1 cup wheat bran
1 teaspoon baking soda
1/2 teaspoon ground cinnamon
1 cup mashed banana
1/4 cup canola oil
1/2 cup light brown sugar
1 large egg
1/2 cup chopped walnuts, optional

Preheat oven to 375 degrees. In a bowl, mix together the flour, wheat bran, baking soda, and cinnamon; set aside. In a mixing bowl, beat together banana and oil. Add the brown sugar and egg, mixing well. Add the dry ingredients, stirring just until blended. Stir in walnuts. Spoon into paper lined muffin tins. Bake 15 minutes.

Nutritional information per serving

Calories 147, Protein (g) 3, Carbohydrate (g) 25, Fat (g) 5, Cal. from Fat (%) 31, Saturated Fat (g) 1, Dietary Fiber (g) 3, Cholesterol (mg) 18, Sodium (mg) 114, Diabetic Exchanges: 1 starch, 0.5 fruit, 1 fat

DOC'S NOTES:

Good breakfast choice.

CONSTIPATION

Lemon Berry Bread 🥕 ❄️

Lemon and berries join together to make this bread a real winner. When blueberries are not in season, leave them out for a delicious lemon bread.

MAKES 16 SERVINGS

1/3 cup canola oil
2/3 cup sugar
2 tablespoons lemon extract
4 large egg whites
1 1/2 cups all-purpose flour
1 teaspoon baking powder
1/2 cup skim milk
1 cup fresh blueberries
2 tablespoons grated lemon rind

Preheat oven to 350 degrees. In a large bowl, mix oil, sugar, lemon extract, and egg whites. In another bowl, combine flour with baking powder. Add flour mixture to sugar mixture alternately with milk, stirring just until blended. Fold in blueberries and lemon rind. Pour batter into a 9×5×3-inch loaf pan coated with nonstick cooking spray and dusted with flour. Bake for 40 to 50 minutes or until a wooden toothpick inserted in center comes out clean. Immediately poke holes at 1-inch intervals into the top of the bread and pour Lemon Glaze (recipe follows) over.

LEMON GLAZE

1/2 cup sugar
1/2 cup lemon juice

In a small saucepan, combine sugar and lemon juice, heating until sugar is dissolved.

Nutritional information per serving
Calories 158, Protein (g) 3, Carbohydrate (g) 26, Fat (g) 5, Cal. from Fat (%) 26, Saturated Fat (g) 0, Dietary Fiber (g) 1, Cholesterol (mg) 0, Sodium (mg) 49, Diabetic Exchanges: 1 starch, 1 other carb., 1 fat

DOC'S NOTES:

Blueberries are an excellent source of antioxidants.

Easy Cranberry Yam Bread 🥕 ❄️

This simple to make bread with the natural sweetness of yams and tartness of cranberries is great to have on hand.

MAKES 16 SLICES

1 (8-ounce) package reduced-fat cream cheese, softened

3/4 cup sugar

1 (15-ounce) can sweet potatoes (yams), drained and mashed

2 large eggs

1 1/2 cups biscuit baking mix

1 teaspoon ground cinnamon

1/2 teaspoon ground nutmeg

1 cup dried cranberries, or chopped fresh cranberries

Preheat oven to 350 degrees. In a mixing bowl, cream together the cream cheese and sugar until light and fluffy. Beat in the sweet potatoes and eggs. Stir in the baking mix, cinnamon, nutmeg, and cranberries until just blended. Pour into a 9×5×3-inch loaf pan coated with nonstick cooking spray. Bake for 45 minutes to 1 hour, or until a toothpick inserted in the center comes out clean. Cool in the pan for 15 minutes.

Nutrition information per serving

Calories 172, Protein (g) 3, Carbohydrate (g) 28, Fat (g) 5, Calories from Fat (%) 28, Saturated Fat (g) 3, Dietary Fiber (g) 1, Cholesterol (mg) 36, Sodium (mg) 215, Diabetic Exchanges: 2 starch, 0.5 fat

CONSTIPATION

Oatmeal Chocolate Cake 🥕 ❄

This moist cake with chocolate laced through makes a great snack. For a chocolate spice cake version, leave out the chocolate chips and add 1 teaspoon cinnamon and 1/2 teaspoon allspice.

MAKES 24 SQUARES

1 1/2 cups boiling water
1 cup old-fashioned oatmeal
1 cup light brown sugar
1/2 cup sugar
1/4 cup canola oil
1/3 cup buttermilk
1 large egg
2 large egg whites
1 teaspoon vanilla extract
1 1/2 cups all-purpose flour
1 teaspoon baking soda
1 tablespoon cocoa
1/2 cup semisweet chocolate chips

Preheat oven to 350 degrees. Coat a 13×9×2-inch baking pan with nonstick cooking spray. Pour the boiling water over the oatmeal in a bowl; let stand for 10 minutes. Add the brown sugar, sugar, oil, and buttermilk, stirring well. Add the egg, egg whites, and vanilla, mixing well. In another bowl, combine the flour, baking soda, and cocoa. Add the dry ingredients to the sugar mixture, mixing well. Stir in the chocolate chips. Pour batter into pan and bake for about 30 minutes. Let cool in pan.

Nutritional information per serving
Calories 135, Protein (g) 2, Carbohydrate (g) 24, Fat (g) 4, Cal. from Fat (%) 25, Saturated Fat (g) 1, Dietary Fiber (g) 1, Cholesterol (mg) 9, Sodium (mg) 68, Diabetic Exchanges: 0.5 starch, 1 other carb., 0.5 fat

DOC'S NOTES:

The oatmeal provides a great source of fiber and will also help lower cholesterol.

Peach Crumble

The crumbly cereal oatmeal topping adds fiber and crunch to this luscious baked peach dessert, which is hard to resist out of the oven. Great served warm with frozen vanilla yogurt for a treat. Any fruit, fresh or frozen, may be substituted for the peaches.

MAKES 6 TO 8 SERVINGS

1/3 cup light brown sugar

3/4 cup old fashioned oatmeal

1/2 cup natural wheat and barley cereal

1/2 cup all-purpose flour

1 1/2 teaspoons ground cinnamon, divided

1/2 teaspoon vanilla extract

2 tablespoons canola oil

2 tablespoons orange juice

1 (16-ounce) package frozen peaches

3 tablespoons sugar

1 tablespoon cornstarch

Preheat the oven to 350 degrees. In a bowl, combine the brown sugar, oatmeal, cereal, flour, and 1/2 teaspoon cinnamon. Stir in the vanilla, canola oil, and orange juice until crumbly; set aside. In a 2-quart dish coated with nonstick cooking spray, toss the peaches with the sugar, remaining 1 teaspoon cinnamon, and cornstarch, coating well. Sprinkle the oatmeal mixture on top. Bake for 35 to 45 minutes or until bubbly.

Nutrition information per serving

Calories 198, Protein (g) 3, Carbohydrate (g) 37, Fat (g) 5, Calories from Fat (%) 21, Saturated Fat (g) 0, Dietary Fiber (g) 3, Cholesterol (mg) 0, Sodium (mg) 48, Diabetic Exchanges: 1 starch, 0.5 fruit, 1 other carbohydrate, 1 fat

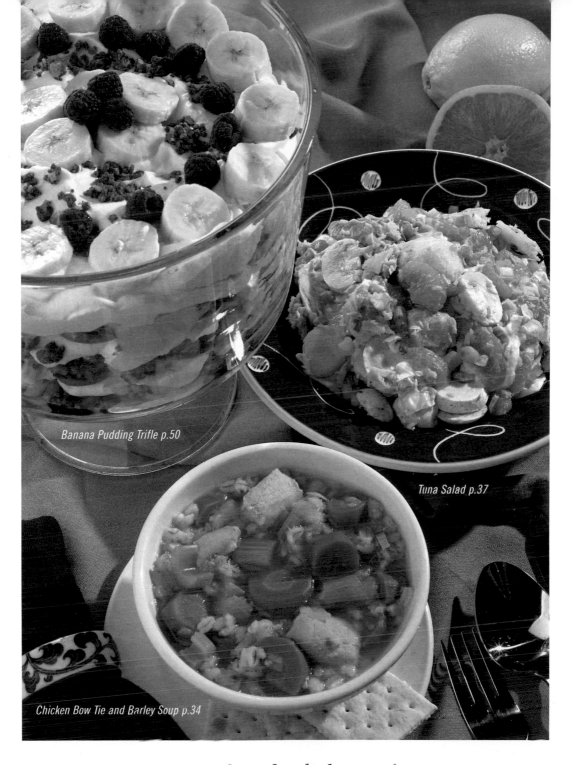

Banana Pudding Trifle p.50

Tuna Salad p.37

Chicken Bow Tie and Barley Soup p.34

Eat a low-fat, light meal
prior to a *Day of Chemotherapy*.

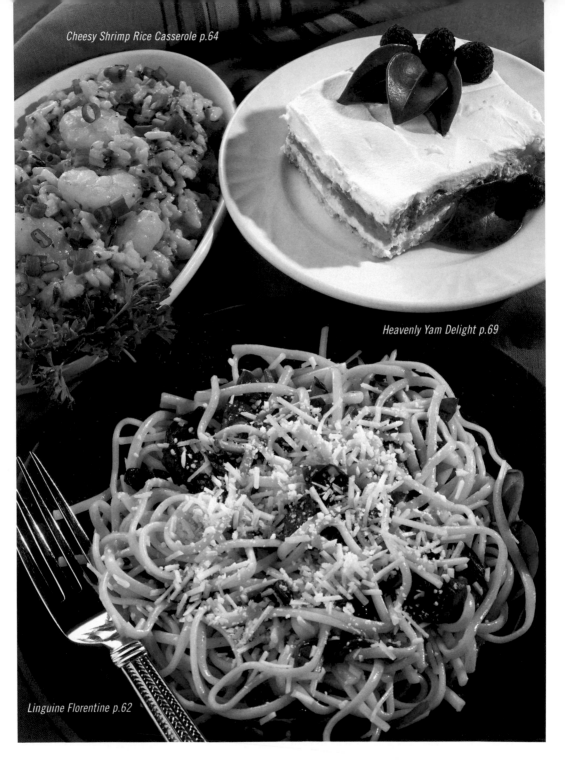

Cheesy Shrimp Rice Casserole p.64

Heavenly Yam Delight p.69

Linguine Florentine p.62

Avoid uncooked fruits, vegetables,
meat, and seafood when *Neutropenic*.

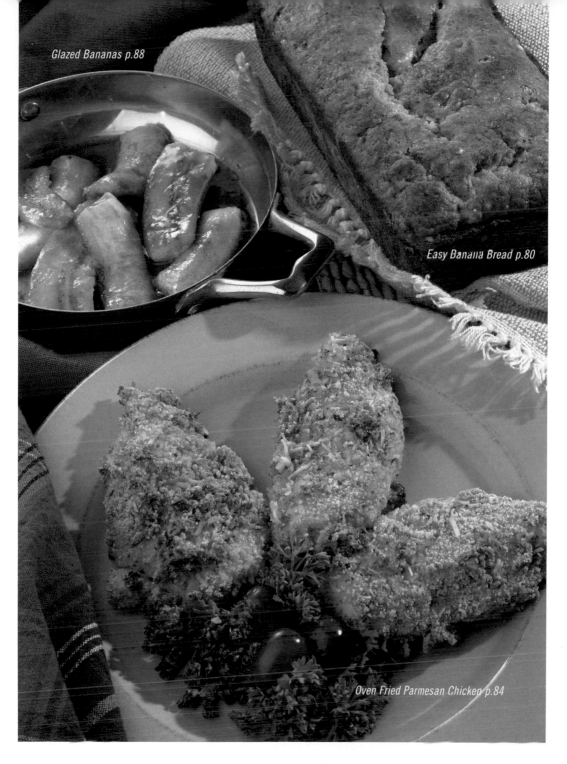

Glazed Bananas p.88

Easy Banana Bread p.80

Oven Fried Parmesan Chicken p.84

Bananas, rice, applesauce, and toast are good foods
when you experience *Diarrhea*.

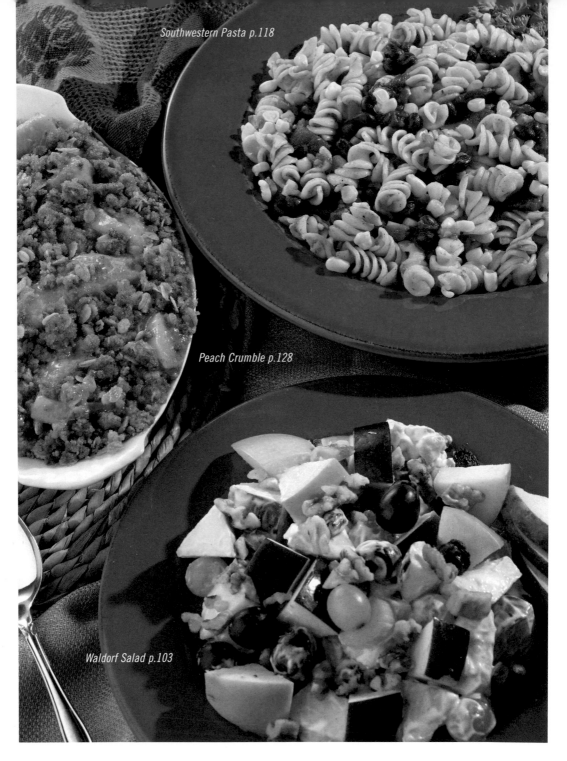

Southwestern Pasta p.118

Peach Crumble p.128

Waldorf Salad p.103

Recipes including fruit and vegetable dishes
should be prepared to eat for *Constipation*.

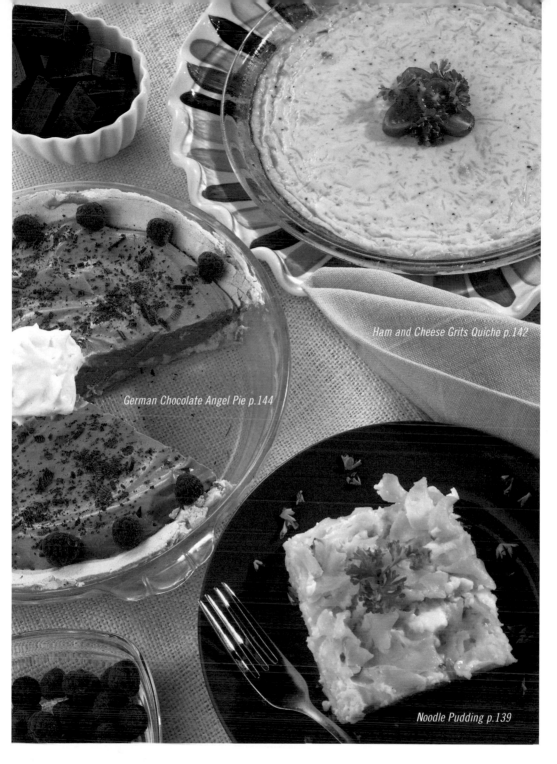

Ham and Cheese Grits Quiche p.142

German Chocolate Angel Pie p.144

Noodle Pudding p.139

Eating soft, bland foods and lukewarm or cold foods can be soothing if you have a *Sore Mouth or Throat*.

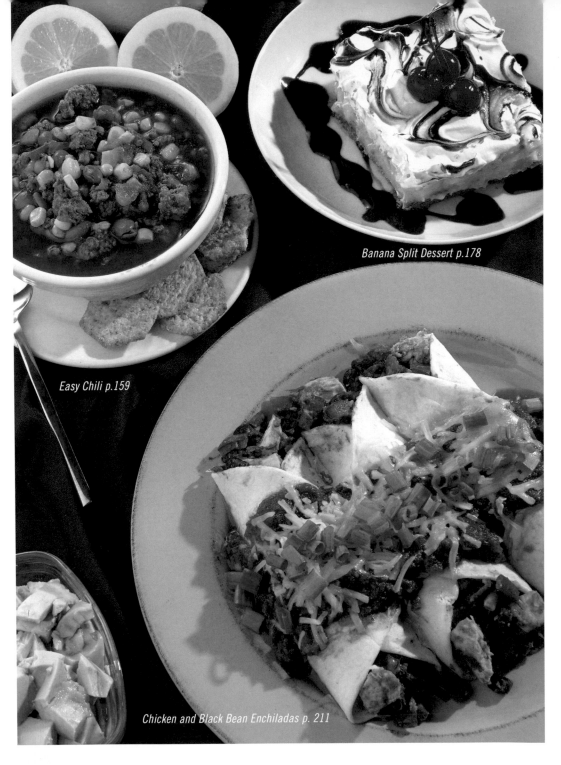

Banana Split Dessert p.178

Easy Chili p.159

Chicken and Black Bean Enchiladas p. 211

High Calorie-High Protein foods help cancer patients maintain their weight and a good nutritional state.

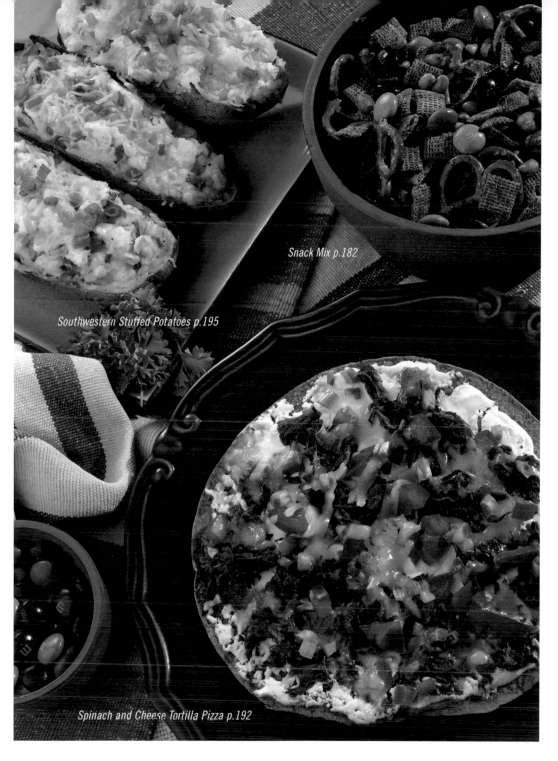

Snack Mix p.182

Southwestern Stuffed Potatoes p.195

Spinach and Cheese Tortilla Pizza p.192

Snacks and Light Meals are important
to help maintain weight.

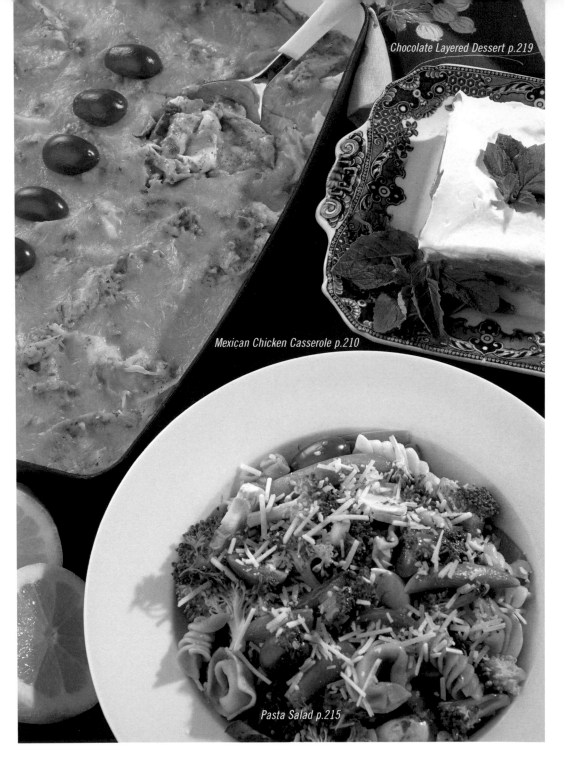

Chocolate Layered Dessert p.219

Mexican Chicken Casserole p.210

Pasta Salad p.215

Food gifts bring joy and happiness to
loved ones and *Caregivers* alike.

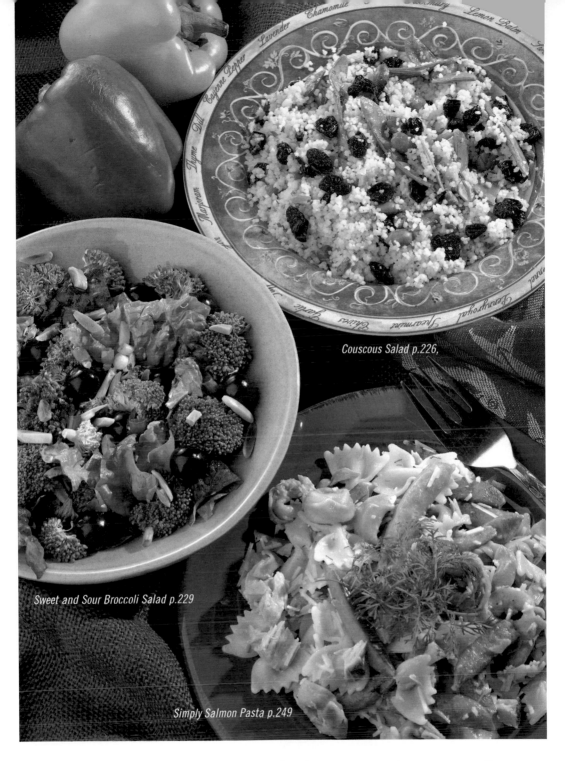

Couscous Salad p.226,

Sweet and Sour Broccoli Salad p.229

Simply Salmon Pasta p.249

The good foods, such as whole grains, legumes, fruits, and vegetables, provide *Healthy Eating Post Treatment.*

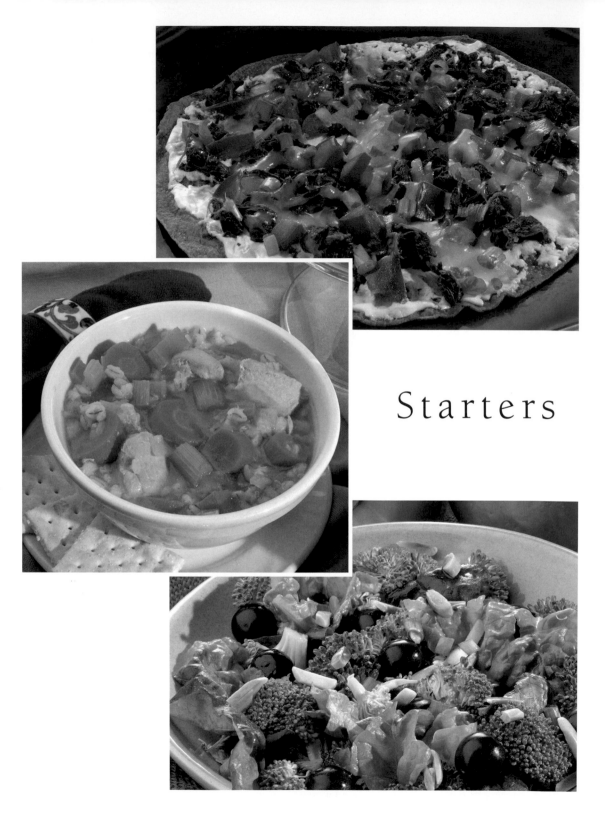

Starters

Spinach and Cheese Tortilla Pizza p. 192; Chicken, Barley and Bow-Tie Soup p. 34; Sweet and Sour Broccoli Salad p. 229

Starters

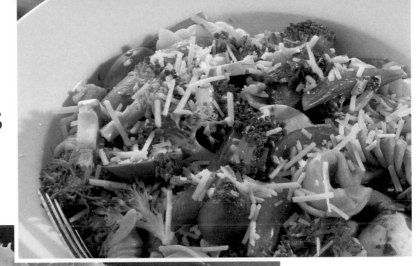

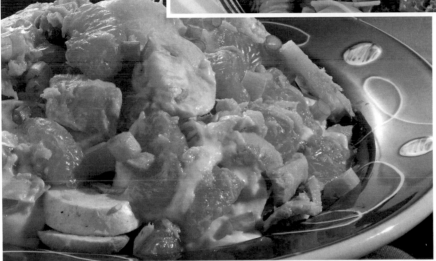

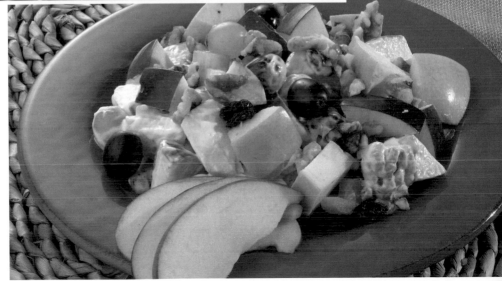

Pasta Salad p. 215; Tuna Salad p. 37; Waldorf Salad p. 103

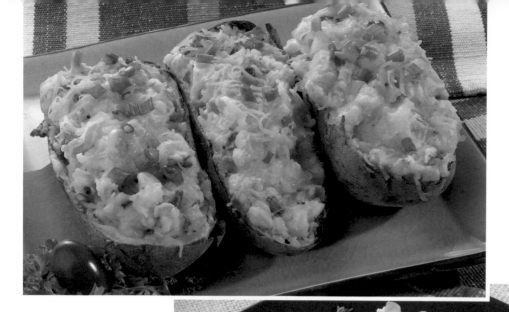

Sides

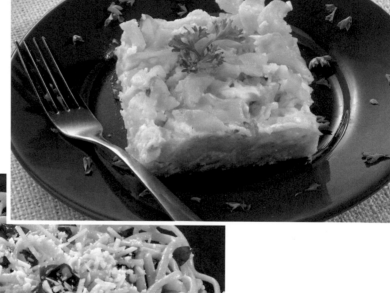

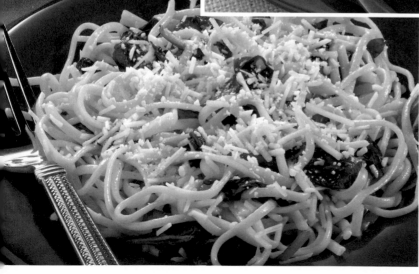

Southwestern Stuffed Potatoes p. 195; Noodle Pudding p. 139; Linguine Florentine p. 62

Entrées

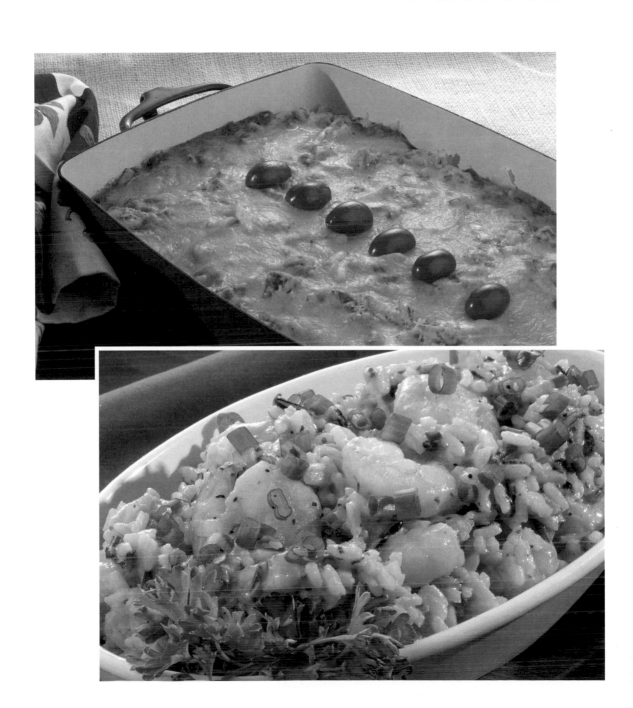

Mexican Chicken Casserole p. 210, Cheesy Shrimp and Rice p. 64

Entrées

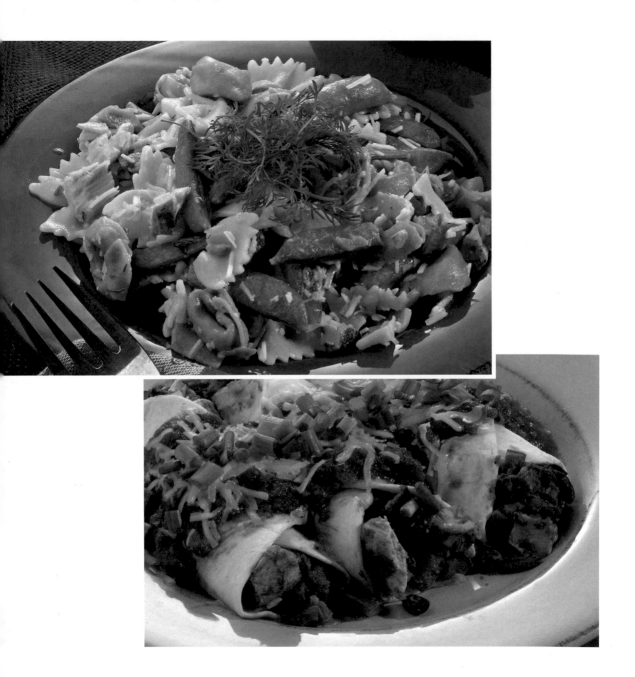

Simply Salmon Pasta p. 249; Chicken and Black Bean Enchiladas, p. 211

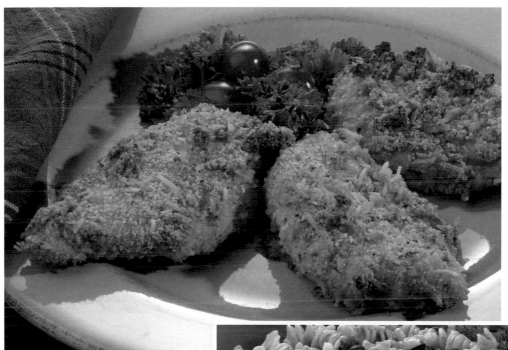

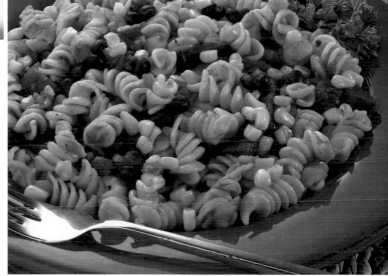

Entrées

Oven Fried Parmesan Chicken, p. 84; Southwestern Pasta, p. 118

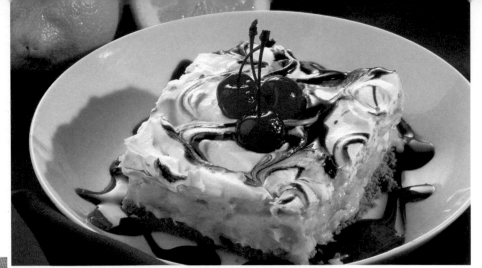

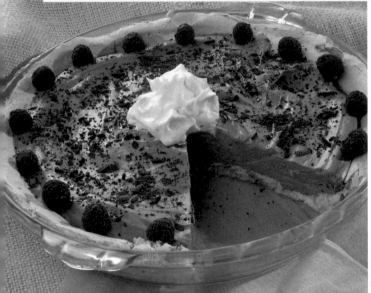

Desserts

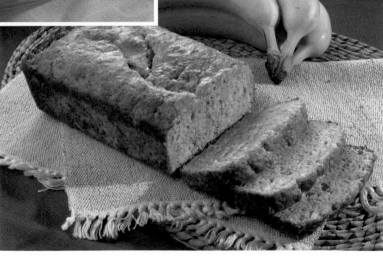

Banana Split Dessert, p. 178; German Chocolate Angel Pie, p. 144; Easy Banana Bread, p. 80

Sore Mouth or Throat

- ✦ I have no appetite. Is there anything to help me?
- ✦ Should I eat hot or cold foods?
- ✦ What foods should I eat?

Your mouth normally will get sore 7 to 10 days following certain chemotherapy treatments. Remember to do your mouth care: 1 teaspoon baking soda, 1 teaspoon salt in a quart of tap water. Rinse and spit after each meal. Make a fresh solution each morning and discard at the end of the day. Try eating soft or puréed foods. Use a straw for all liquids or puréed foods. This is a good time to use plastic utensils to avoid the metallic taste. Eating foods at room temperature or cool are easier to handle when your mouth is sore. Raw foods tend to irritate your mouth and should be avoided. If you are still losing ground, talk to your physicians about the following appetite stimulants:

1—Liquid Megace – 800 mg/day x 30 days then decrease to 400 mg/day.
2—Megace 40 mg twice per day and Marinol 2.5 mg by mouth twice per day.

Remember, if you find one food that you can tolerate do not hesitate to eat it repeatedly. The mouth soreness is usually associated with a low white blood cell count. As soon as your counts rise, the soreness will resolve. Cephacol, Xylocaine, and pain medicines are sometimes needed to ease the mouth pain. I often have patients take a pain pill 30 minutes prior to meals to allow them to eat. If you have obvious sores on your lips, a small amount of Vitamin E can sometimes help. Puncture a 500 unit Vitamin E capsule and squeeze the contents on the ulcer 3 times per day.

If you have these problems, eating soft, bland foods and lukewarm or cool foods can be soothing. On the other hand, foods that are coarse, dry, or scratchy should be avoided. In addition, you may find that tart, salty or acidic fruits and juices, alcohol, and spicy foods may be irritating and should be avoided. Rinsing your mouth regularly with one teaspoon of baking soda and eight ounces of water or salt water can help prevent infections and improve healing.

Points To Remember
- ✦ Avoid tart, acidic, or salty foods and drinks such as citrus fruit juices (grapefruit, orange, lime), pickled and vinegary foods, tomato-based foods, and some canned broths.
- ✦ Avoid rough-textured foods, such as dry toast, granola, and raw fruits and vegetables.
- ✦ Eat food that is cool or room temperature. Very hot or cold foods can cause discomfort.

- Limit alcohol, caffeine, and tobacco. These substances can dry out your mouth and throat and promote further irritation.
- Avoid spices such as chili powder, cloves, curry, hot sauces, nutmeg, and pepper.
- Season foods with herbs such as basil, oregano, and thyme.
- Use a straw for liquids.
- Try chewing sugar-free gum or suck on sugar free candies.
- Cut food into small pieces.
- Softer and easy to swallow foods include soft, creamy foods such as cream soups, cheeses, mashed potatoes, pastas, yogurt, eggs, custards, puddings, cooked cereals, ice cream, casseroles, gravies, syrups, breakfast-type recipes, milkshakes, and nutritional liquid food supplements.
- Drink your meals with nutritious liquids.
- Practice good oral hygiene.
- Use oral anesthetics such as ulcerease. Ask your doctor for a "stomatitis (sore mouth) cocktail."
  Xylocaine—equal parts; Maalox—equal parts; Benadryl—equal parts
  Swish and swallow one teaspoon every four hours as needed for pain.

Some Soft Foods to Include:
- Applesauce, bananas, watermelon, and other soft fruits.
- Cottage cheese, milk shakes, or smoothies. Scrambled eggs.
- Puddings, flavored gelatin. Cooked cereals such as oatmeal or cream of wheat.
- Mashed potatoes or sweet potatoes, macaroni and cheese, or mashed vegetables.

Shopping List for Sore Mouth
- Bread, butter, eggs, honey
- Cream of wheat, grits
- Applesauce; fruit, no citrus (fresh, frozen, canned); vegetables (fresh, frozen, canned)
- Milk, cottage cheese, ice cream, frozen yogurt, cheese, yogurt
- Nutritional energy drink supplement
- Popsicles, puddings, flavored gelatins, frozen whipped topping

Menus

Foods to eat when sore mouth or throat is occurring.

Breakfast

25   Baked French Toast
Banana

28   Egg Soufflé

56   Quick Cheese Grits

134   Applesauce Oatmeal

142   Ham and Cheese Grits Quiche
Soft fruits such as watermelon, papaya

Lunch

32   Asparagus and Potato Soup
Grilled Cheese Sandwich
Applesauce

136   Avocado Soup

193   Cheese Quesadillas

198   Mocha Meringue Mounds

Dinner

Quick Shrimp Sauté   143
Creamed Double Potatoes   141
Cream Cheese Bread Pudding   145

Veggie Plate

Carrot Soufflé   140
Cheesy Macaroni   40
Lemon Angel Food Cake   51

Bread Pudding Florentine   27
Quick Cheese Grits   56
Mock Chocolate Éclair   52

Snacks

Strawberry Weight Gain Shake   146
Spinach Dip   184
German Chocolate Angel Pie   144
Sweet Potato Shake   136
Cantaloupe Banana Smoothie   136
Awesome Milk Shake   146

Melon Soup 🥕

A cool, refreshing soup or can be served in a glass for a great drink.

MAKES 2 SERVINGS

3 cups cubed cantaloupe
1 tablespoon lime juice
1 teaspoon sugar
1 cup nonfat plain yogurt
1 teaspoon vanilla extract

Mix together all ingredients in a food processor; process until smooth.

Nutritional information per serving
Calories 169, Protein (g) 9, Carbohydrate (g) 33,
Fat (g) 1, Cal. from Fat (%) 5, Saturated Fat (g) 0,
Dietary Fiber (g) 2, Cholesterol (mg) 2, Sodium (mg) 116,
Diabetic Exchanges: 1.5 fruit, 1 skim milk

DOC'S NOTES:

Sip through a straw until it is all gone.
Great source of potassium.

Simple Vichyssoise ❄️

The longer it sits the better it gets! Use reduced-sodium chicken broth to reduce the sodium.

MAKES 8 SERVINGS

3½ cups canned fat-free chicken broth
2 (10½-ounce) cans cream of potato soup
2 cups nonfat plain yogurt
⅓ cup chopped green onions (scallions), optional

In a bowl, combine broth, soup, and yogurt, mixing well. Refrigerate for several hours. Sprinkle with green onions when serving.

Nutritional information per serving
Calories 86, Protein (g) 6, Carbohydrate (g) 12,
Fat (g) 2, Cal. from Fat (%) 16, Saturated Fat (g) 1,
Dietary Fiber (g) 0, Cholesterol (mg) 5, Sodium (mg) 926,
Diabetic Exchanges: 0.5 starch, 0.5 skim milk

DOC'S NOTES:

Good source of protein, potassium and complex carbs.

SORE MOUTH OR THROAT

Weight Gain Pancakes 🥕

Top with fresh fruit or sliced bananas for added nutrition. Whole milk can be used instead of the supplement, if desired.

MAKES 6 TO 7 PANCAKES

1/2 cup pancake and waffle mix
1/2 cup vanilla nutritional energy drink
  supplement
1 large egg
1 tablespoon canola oil

Preheat griddle to 400 degrees or until drops of water sizzle then evaporate on griddle. Combine all ingredients and mix with a wire whip or fork until fairly smooth. Do not overmix as this will cause thin, tough pancakes. Let batter stand 1 to 2 minutes. Pour a scant 1/4 cup of batter for each pancake onto a lightly greased griddle. Turn pancakes when edges look cooked and tops are covered with bubbles. Turn only once.

Nutritional information per serving

Calories 80, Protein (g) 3, Carbohydrate (g) 10, Fat (g) 3, Cal. from Fat (%) 39, Saturated Fat (g) 1, Dietary Fiber (g) 0, Cholesterol (mg) 32, Sodium (mg) 131, Diabetic Exchanges: 0.5 starch, 0.5 fat

DOC'S NOTES:

The nutritional energy drink supplement supplies essential vitamins and minerals, plus high quality protein and carbs for energy, making it a great way to use as added value for milk in recipes.

Applesauce Oatmeal ✎

Great way to start off your day as this recipe takes oatmeal to a new level. Instead of applesauce, try stirring in a mashed banana for banana oatmeal and, if your mouth isn't sore, add some raisins.

MAKES TWO (3/4-CUP) SERVINGS

1 cup skim milk
3/4 cup old fashioned oatmeal
1/2 cup unsweetened applesauce
1 tablespoon light brown sugar
1/8 teaspoon ground cinnamon

In a small saucepan, bring milk to a boil. Add the oatmeal and reduce heat. Cook for about 5 minutes or until thickened, stirring occasionally. Add the applesauce, brown sugar, and cinnamon, stirring until well mixed. Serve immediately.

Nutritional information per serving

Calories 212, Protein (g) 9, Carbohydrate (g) 40, Fat (g) 2, Cal. from Fat (%) 9, Saturated Fat (g) 1, Dietary Fiber (g) 4, Cholesterol (mg) 2, Sodium (mg) 68, Diabetic Exchanges: 1.5 starch, 0.5 fruit, 0.5 skim milk, 0.5 other carb.

DOC'S NOTES:

The oatmeal provides fiber while the applesauce provides vitamin C and beta-carotene.

Watermelon Slush 🥕

Great source of potassium and Vitamin C.

MAKES 2 SERVINGS

1 cup of ice
3 cups watermelon chunks
2 tablespoons honey

Blend all ingredients in a blender or food processor.

Nutritional information per serving

Calories 137, Protein (g) 2, Carbohydrate (g) 34, Fat (g) 1, Cal. from Fat (%) 6, Saturated Fat (g) 0, Dietary Fiber (g) 1, Cholesterol (mg) 0, Sodium (mg) 5, Diabetic Exchanges: 1 fruit, 1 other carb.

DOC'S NOTES:

For cancer patients, watermelon seems to be the most tolerated fruit. It's light, cool, refreshing and goes down easy.

Cantaloupe Banana Smoothie 🥕

Fruits team up for a nutritious smoothie — potassium plus!

MAKES 2 SERVINGS

1 teaspoon vanilla extract
1 banana
1 cup cubed cantaloupe
1 tablespoon honey
1 cup reduced-fat vanilla ice cream

Blend all ingredients in a blender or food processor until smooth.

Nutritional information per serving

Calories 231, Protein (g) 4, Carbohydrate (g) 49, Fat (g) 3, Cal. from Fat (%) 9, Saturated Fat (g) 1, Dietary Fiber (g) 3, Cholesterol (mg) 5, Sodium (mg) 53, Diabetic Exchanges: 1.5 fruit, 2 other carb., 0.5 fat

DOC'S NOTES:

For extra calories and nutrition, substitute vanilla nutritional drink supplement for ice cream.

Sweet Potato Shake

Packed full of nutrition. Serve cold!

MAKES 2 SERVINGS

1/2 cup mashed cooked sweet potatoes (yams)
1 (12-ounce) can apricot nectar, chilled
2 tablespoons honey
1/2 teaspoon vanilla extract

Using a food processor, blend all ingredients until smooth. Refrigerate.

Nutritional information per serving

Calories 255, Protein (g) 2, Carbohydrate (g) 64,
Fat (g) 0, Cal. from Fat (%) 0, Saturated Fat (g) 0,
Dietary Fiber (g) 3, Cholesterol (mg) 0, Sodium (mg) 17,
Diabetic Exchanges: 1.5 starch, 1.5 fruit, 1 other carb.

DOC'S NOTES:

Rich in beta carotene and Vitamins C and B.

Avocado Soup

This marvelous rich, creamy soup is a great source of monounsaturated fats. If clam juice is not available, use extra chicken broth.

MAKES 4 SERVINGS

2 large avocados, peeled and pit removed
1 teaspoon minced garlic
2 cups canned fat-free chicken broth
1 (8-ounce) bottle clam juice
1/2 cup nonfat plain yogurt

Using a food processor, blend all ingredients until smooth. Refrigerate.

Nutritional information per serving

Calories 198, Protein (g) 6, Carbohydrate (g) 13,
Fat (g) 16, Cal. from Fat (%) 65, Saturated Fat (g) 3,
Dietary Fiber (g) 9, Cholesterol (mg) 1, Sodium (mg) 734,
Diabetic Exchanges: 1 fruit, 3 fat

DOC'S NOTES:

Use more chicken broth for the clam juice to reduce the sodium.

Cream of Spinach and Brie Soup 🥕

Sneak spinach into your diet with this wonderful creamy soup. Try using Swiss chard for spinach to include a cruciferous vegetable. This is a little high in saturated fat but perfect to entice your appetite. I couldn't leave this recipe out.

MAKES 6 SERVINGS

1/2 cup chopped onion

1/3 cup all-purpose flour

2 cups skim milk

2 cups chicken broth

8 ounces Brie cheese, rind removed and cubed

2 cups fresh spinach, washed and stemmed

Salt and pepper to taste

In a nonstick pot coated with nonstick cooking spray, sauté onion until soft. Stir in flour. Gradually stir in milk and chicken broth. Bring to a boil over medium heat, stirring constantly, until thickened. Add cheese and stir until melted. Add spinach and salt and pepper, stirring until spinach is wilted.

Nutritional information per serving
Calories 192, Protein (g) 13, Carbohydrate (g) 11, Fat (g) 11, Cal. from Fat (%) 50, Saturated Fat (g) 7, Dietary Fiber (g) 1, Cholesterol (mg) 39, Sodium (mg) 495, Diabetic Exchanges: 1 high fat meat, 0.5 starch, 0.5 skim milk

DOC'S NOTES:

Spinach is a great source of iron, Vitamin A, and calcium. Iron is essential to the formation of hemoglobin, which carries oxygen in the blood, and myoglobin, which carries oxygen in muscle.

Baked Acorn Squash 🥕

When this winter squash is in season, here is an easy very tasty recipe. Just adjust the amounts of sugar and margarine for how many squash you are preparing.

MAKES 2 SERVINGS

1 large acorn squash
2 tablespoons light brown sugar
2 teaspoons margarine

Preheat oven to 350 degrees. Cut squash in half and scoop out seeds and strings; discard. Place in a baking dish filled with 1/2-inch water, open side up. Bake for 40 minutes. Remove from oven and fill each half with 1 tablespoon brown sugar and 1 teaspoon margarine. Return to oven and continue baking for 10 minutes longer or until tender.

Nutritional information per serving

Calories 172, Protein (g) 2, Carbohydrate (g) 36, Fat (g) 4, Cal. from Fat (%) 19, Saturated Fat (g) 1, Dietary Fiber (g) 3, Cholesterol (mg) 0, Sodium (mg) 56, Diabetic Exchanges: 1.5 starch, 1 other carb., 1 fat

DOC'S NOTES:

Excellent source of calcium and beta carotene. One cup of acorn squash supplies 90mg of calcium — 11% of the recommended daily allowance.

Noodle Pudding ❄

A plain, slightly sweet dish that makes a nice side dish.

MAKES 15 SERVINGS

1 (8-ounce) package wide noodles
4 tablespoons margarine, melted
1/2 cup sugar
1 cup low fat cottage cheese
1 (8-ounce) container nonfat plain yogurt
4 ounces light cream cheese
3 large egg whites
1/2 teaspoon vanilla extract

Preheat oven to 350 degrees. Boil noodles according to directions on package, omitting oil. Rinse, drain, and combine with margarine, tossing evenly. Place noodles in a glass 13×9×2-inch baking pan coated with nonstick cooking spray. In food processor or mixer, combine remaining ingredients, beating until smooth. Combine with noodles, mixing well. Bake for 45 to 60 minutes.

Nutritional information per serving

Calories 150, Protein (g) 6, Carbohydrate (g) 20, Fat (g) 5, Cal. from Fat (%) 30, Saturated Fat (g) 2, Dietary Fiber (g) 0, Cholesterol (mg) 20, Sodium (mg) 147, Diabetic Exchanges: 0.5 very lean meat, 1 starch, 0.5 other carb., 1 fat

DOC'S NOTES:

Excellent source of protein and calcium.

Carrot Soufflé 🥕 ❄

Carrots will never have tasted so good!!
Adjust sugar for a less sweet version.

MAKES 8 SERVINGS

2 pounds carrots, sliced
1/3 cup sugar
2 large egg whites
3 large eggs
2 tablespoons all-purpose flour
1 1/2 teaspoons baking powder
3 tablespoons margarine, softened
1 teaspoon vanilla extract

Preheat oven to 350 degrees. Cook carrots in a small amount of water or in the microwave until very soft; drain well. In a mixing bowl, beat carrots. Add sugar, egg whites, and eggs. Mix together flour and baking powder, and add to carrot mixture, blending well. Add margarine and vanilla. Transfer to an oblong baking dish coated with nonstick cooking spray and bake for 1 hour.

Nutritional information per serving
Calories 157, Protein (g) 5, Carbohydrate (g) 21,
Fat (g) 6, Cal. from Fat (%) 36, Saturated Fat (g) 1,
Dietary Fiber (g) 3, Cholesterol (mg) 79, Sodium (mg) 219,
Diabetic Exchanges: 3 vegetable, 0.5 other carb., 1 fat

DOC'S NOTES:

Carrots are high in Vitamin C, beta carotene, and potassium. They are also a good source of fiber.

Creamed Double Potatoes ✎ ❄

Sweet potatoes are rich in beta carotene and vitamins. This will be easy to tolerate and you are getting valuable nutrition.

MAKES 8 SERVINGS

1³/4 pounds baking potatoes
1³/4 pounds sweet potatoes (yams)
3 tablespoons margarine
1/3 cup skim milk
2 tablespoons honey

In large pot, cover both types of potatoes with water and boil for 40 minutes or until tender. Peel potatoes and place in mixing bowl with the margarine, blending until smooth. Gradually add the milk and honey, beating until creamy.

Nutritional information per serving

Calories 240, Protein (g) 4, Carbohydrate (g) 47, Fat (g) 5, Cal. from Fat (%) 17, Saturated Fat (g) 1, Dietary Fiber (g) 5, Cholesterol (mg) 0, Sodium (mg) 74, Diabetic Exchanges: 3 starch, 1 fat

DOC'S NOTES:

Potatoes are rich in Vitamins B6, C, iron, magnesium, niacin, and potassium. Sweet potatoes provide Vitamins A, B6, and C.

Ham and Cheese Grits Quiche

Depending on how you feel, be creative with this very tasty recipe by adding sautéed veggies of your choice. This quiche is a nice change for breakfast or for a light meal.

MAKES 6 SERVINGS

1 cup water

1/3 cup dry quick-cooking grits

1 cup evaporated skim milk

1 cup shredded reduced-fat sharp
  Cheddar cheese

1/2 cup finely diced ham

2 large eggs

2 large egg whites

Salt and pepper to taste

Dash of Worcestershire sauce

Preheat oven to 350 degrees. In a small saucepan, bring the water to a boil; stir in grits. Reduce heat, cover, and cook about 5 minutes or until slightly thickened. In a bowl, combine cooked grits, milk, cheese, ham, eggs, egg whites, salt and pepper, and Worcestershire sauce. Pour mixture into a 9-inch pie plate coated with nonstick cooking spray. Bake for 30 minutes or until set.

Nutritional information per serving

Calories 172, Protein (g) 16, Carbohydrate (g) 12, Fat (g) 6, Cal. from Fat (%) 33, Saturated Fat (g) 3, Dietary Fiber (g) 0, Cholesterol (mg) 93, Sodium (mg) 216, Diabetic Exchanges: 2 lean meat, 0.5 starch, 0.5 skim milk

DOC'S NOTES:

This tasty breakfast dish is a good source of calories and protein and can be enjoyed all day long.

Quick Shrimp Sauté

In the mood for an easy yet delicious shrimp dish? Serve over rice or pasta.

MAKES 6 SERVINGS

2 TABLESPOONS MARGARINE

1 bunch green onions (scallions),
  chopped, optional
1 teaspoon minced garlic
2 pounds medium shrimp, peeled
1 tablespoon Worcestershire sauce
1 teaspoon dried basil leaves
2 cups nonfat plain yogurt
1 tablespoon all-purpose flour

In a large skillet, melt the margarine and sauté the green onions and garlic for two minutes. Add the shrimp, Worcestershire sauce, and basil, cooking until the shrimp are done, about 5 to 7 minutes. Mix the yogurt with the flour and stir into the shrimp mixture and heat thoroughly; do not boil.

Nutritional information per serving
Calories 184, Protein (g) 25, Carbohydrate (g) 9, Fat (g) 5, Cal. from Fat (%) 25, Saturated Fat (g) 1, Dietary Fiber (g) 1, Cholesterol (mg) 181, Sodium (mg) 344, Diabetic Exchanges: 3 very lean meat, 0.5 skim milk, 0.5 fat

DOC'S NOTES:

This can be chopped or puréed to make it easier to eat.

German Chocolate Angel Pie 🥕 ❄

Easy, refreshing fabulous dessert, make ahead and freeze. Easy to swallow as it melts in your mouth.

MAKES 8 SERVINGS

3 large egg whites, room temperature
¼ teaspoon salt
¼ teaspoon cream of tartar
¾ cup sugar
1 tablespoon plus 1 teaspoon vanilla extract, divided
1 (4-ounce) bar German Sweet Chocolate
3 tablespoons water
1 (8-ounce) container fat-free frozen whipped topping, thawed

Preheat oven to 300 degrees. Beat egg whites with salt and cream of tartar until foamy. Add sugar, 2 tablespoons at a time, beating well after each addition. Continue beating until stiff peaks form. Fold in 1 tablespoon vanilla. Spoon into 9-inch lightly greased glass pie plate and form nest-like shell. Bake 45 minutes. Cool. In a microwave safe bowl, melt chocolate in water for 1 minute, stir until melted. Cool. Add remaining 1 teaspoon vanilla. Fold whipped topping into cooled chocolate. Spoon into meringue shell. Freeze. Thaw slightly to serve.

Nutritional information per serving
Calories 198, Protein (g) 2, Carbohydrate (g) 37, Fat (g) 4, Cal. from Fat (%) 17, Saturated Fat (g) 2, Dietary Fiber (g) 1, Cholesterol (mg) 0, Sodium (mg) 109, Diabetic Exchanges: 2.5 other carb., 1 fat

DOC'S NOTES:

Good source of calories and very soothing for a sore mouth as the crust is a meringue.

Cream Cheese
Bread Pudding 🥕

Bread pudding is always a popular dessert, but with the cream cheese topping it reaches new heights! If having trouble swallowing, use regular bread and cut off the crusts.

MAKES 8 SERVINGS

1 (16-ounce) loaf French bread

2 large eggs, divided

4 large egg whites, divided

1 cup sugar, divided

1 teaspoon vanilla extract

1 teaspoon imitation butter flavoring

3 cups skim milk

1 teaspoon ground cinnamon

1 (8-ounce) package fat-free cream
  cheese, softened

Preheat oven to 350 degrees. Cut the French bread into 1-inch squares. Place the bread in a 13×9×2-inch baking dish. In a large bowl, lightly beat together 1 egg and 3 egg whites. Add 1/2 cup sugar, vanilla, and butter flavoring; mix well. Slowly add the milk to the egg mixture, mixing well. Pour over the bread squares. Sprinkle the mixture with the cinnamon. In a large mixing bowl, beat the cream cheese with the remaining 1/2 cup sugar. Add the remaining egg and egg white, blending until smooth. Spread the mixture evenly over the soaked bread. Bake, uncovered, for 45 minutes or until firm. Let cool slightly before serving.

Nutritional information per serving
Calories 340, Protein (g) 16, Carbohydrate (g) 62, Fat (g) 3, Cal. from Fat (%) 8, Saturated Fat (g) 1, Dietary Fiber (g) 2, Cholesterol (mg) 57, Sodium (mg) 573, Diabetic Exchanges: 1 very lean meat, 2 starch, 0.5 skim milk, 1.5 other carb.

DOC'S NOTES:

Another good source of calcium and protein.

Strawberry Weight Gain Shake 🥕

Try placing the shake in freezer trays. Freeze 1 1/2 hours or serve in a glass and stir until desired consistency.

MAKES 1 SERVING

1 (8-ounce) can vanilla nutritional energy drink
  supplement, chilled
1 cup frozen strawberries (unsweetened)
2 teaspoons sugar

Place supplement and strawberries in a blender. Add sugar and blend until smooth.

Nutritional information per serving

Calories 320, Protein (g) 11, Carbohydrate (g) 62, Fat (g) 4, Cal. from Fat (%) 12, Saturated Fat (g) 0, Dietary Fiber (g) 3, Cholesterol (mg) 0, Sodium (mg) 131, Diabetic Exchanges: 2.5 starch, 1 fruit, 0.5 other carb., 0.5 fat

DOC'S NOTES:

A good source of Vitamin C, potassium, and extra calories. A great way to hide the nutritional supplement.

Awesome Milk Shake 🥕

Try different flavored ice cream for more options.

MAKES 2 SERVINGS

1/2 cup skim milk
2 cups frozen nonfat vanilla yogurt or
  fat-free ice cream
1 teaspoon vanilla extract
3 tablespoons chocolate syrup, optional

In a blender or food processor, place the milk, frozen yogurt, and vanilla and blend until smooth. If you want a chocolate milk shake, add the chocolate syrup to the mixture

Nutritional information per serving

Calories 218, Protein (g) 12, Carbohydrate (g) 41, Fat (g) 0, Cal. from Fat (%) 0, Saturated Fat (g) 0, Dietary Fiber (g) 0, Cholesterol (mg) 4, Sodium (mg) 160, Diabetic Exchanges: 0.5 skim milk, 2.5 other carb.

DOC'S NOTES:

For extra calories, don't use low-fat products and substitute a vanilla nutritional energy drink supplement.

High Calorie-
High Protein

◆ Is weight loss a problem during treatment?

◆ Can your appetite change during the day?

◆ When I don't have an appetite, do I have to eat three large meals per day? If not, what should I do?

◆ Why do I need more protein in my diet?

◆ What are some good sources of protein?

Patients should try to avoid weight loss. Weight loss can be a serious problem for patients undergoing chemotherapy and/or radiation therapy. It has been proven that cancer patients who maintain their weight and maintain a good nutritional state tend to have fewer complications from chemotherapy, radiation therapy or surgery. These patients tend to have shorter hospital stays, reduced illness, fewer infections, have less of a down time and tend to better maintain strength and a sense of well-being.

It is very common for the appetite to decrease as the day progresses. If this occurs, make breakfast your big meal. If you crave or feel you can tolerate a steak and baked potato for breakfast, go for it!

Eating small meals throughout the day is very acceptable. Try eating small, frequent meals and snacks every one to two hours. Keep high-protein, high-calorie snacks and foods handy to eat when you are hungry. If solid foods don't appeal to you, try drinking liquids whenever possible. On the other hand, limit liquids with meals (unless needed to help swallow or for dry mouth) to keep from feeling full early. Avoid food smells when cooking as it can upset the appetite.

There are times that people with cancer need more protein. Protein helps to ensure growth, to repair body tissue, and to maintain a healthy immune system. Without enough protein, the body can take longer to recover from illness and you can have a lower resistance to infection. Following surgery, chemotherapy, and radiation therapy, additional protein is usually needed to heal tissues and to help prevent infection.

Good sources of protein include lean meat, fish, poultry, dairy products, nuts, dried beans, peas and lentils, and soy foods. Fortified milk (recipe included in book) is a great way to add protein to recipes.

Tips for more Calories and Protein

- ✦ Keep snacks handy to have available all the time.
- ✦ Quick and easy snacks include: cheese and crackers, muffins, ice cream, peanut butter, fruit, and pudding are good possibilities.
- ✦ Take a portable snack with you when you go out, such as peanut butter crackers or small boxes of raisins.
- ✦ Even if you don't feel like eating solid foods, try to drink liquids during the day. Juice, soup, and other fluids give you important calories and nutrients. Milk-based drinks also provide protein.
- ✦ For extra protein in dishes, consider adding a little nonfat instant dry milk to scrambled eggs, soup, cereal, sauces, and gravies.
- ✦ Use instant breakfast powder in milk drinks, desserts, ice cream, and milk
- ✦ Try hard-cooked eggs, luncheon meats, peanut butter, cheese, ice cream, granola bars, nutritional supplements, puddings, chips, crackers, and pretzels.

Foods that Provide 7 Grams of Protein Per Serving

- ✦ 1 cup legumes
- ✦ 1 to 2 ounces nuts or seeds
- ✦ 2 tablespoons peanut butter
- ✦ 1 cup rice
- ✦ 1 cup tofu
- ✦ 2.5 ounces tempeh
- ✦ 1 cup cottage cheese
- ✦ 1 ounce cheese
- ✦ 7 ounces milk or yogurt

How to Add Protein and/or Calories to Your Diet
CHEESE

- ✦ Melt on sandwiches, breads, muffins, omelets, tortillas or any meat, chicken or fish.

COTTAGE CHEESE/RICOTTA/CREAM CHEESE

- ✦ Add to casseroles, spaghetti, and pasta.
- ✦ Use as stuffing for crepes, pasta shells, or manicotti.
- ✦ Add to omelets, scrambled eggs, and pancake batter.
- ✦ Spread cream cheese on bread, muffins, fruit and crackers.

SOUR CREAM

+ Add to cream soups, baked potatoes, macaroni and cheese, vegetables, sauces, salad dressings, stews, baked meat, and fish.
+ Use as a topping for cakes, fruit, gelatin desserts, breads, and muffins.
+ Use as a dip for fresh fruits and vegetables.
+ For dessert, scoop it on fresh fruit, add brown sugar, and refrigerate until cold before eating.

EGGS

+ Add chopped hard-boiled eggs to salads, vegetable dishes, and casseroles.
+ Add extra eggs or egg whites to quiches, pancakes, and French toast batter.
+ Add extra eggs or egg whites to scrambled eggs and omelets.
+ Add extra eggs or egg whites to custards and puddings.

MILK

+ Use milk instead of water for liquid when cooking.
+ Use in preparing hot cereal, soups, hot chocolate, and puddings.
+ Use to make cream sauces for vegetables and other recipes.

NONFAT INSTANT DRY MILK

+ Add to milk and milk drinks.
+ Use in casseroles, sauces, cream soups, mashed potatoes, custards and milk-based desserts.

ICE CREAM, YOGURT AND FROZEN YOGURT

+ Add to carbonated beverages, creating ice cream floats.
+ Add to milk drinks like milk shakes.
+ Serve ice cream or yogurt with cake, cookies, graham crackers or any dessert.
+ Make breakfast drinks with fruit and bananas.

SOY

+ Add tofu to shakes and dips.
+ Snack on edamame or add to vegetable dishes, salads, and main dishes.

PEANUT BUTTER

+ Spread on sandwiches, crackers, muffins, pancakes, fruit, and celery.
+ Use as a dip for raw vegetables.

- ✦ Blend with milk drinks.
- ✦ Swirl with ice cream and frozen yogurt.

MEAT AND FISH
- ✦ Add chopped cooked meat or fish to salads, casseroles, soups, and sauces.
- ✦ Use in omelets, quiches, sandwich filling, dressings and stuffings.
- ✦ Add to baked potato.
- ✦ When cooking meat, make a glaze or sauce to cook.

BEANS/LEGUMES
- ✦ Add to soups, casseroles, pastas, and main dishes.

NUTS, SEEDS AND WHEAT GERM
- ✦ Add to casseroles, breads, muffins, pancakes, cookies, and waffles.
- ✦ Sprinkle on fruit, cereal, ice cream, vegetables, salads, and desserts.
- ✦ Roll fruit in nuts.

How to Increase Calories
SALAD DRESSINGS AND MAYONNAISE (INCREASE CALORIES)
- ✦ Use with sandwiches.
- ✦ Combine with meat, fish, and egg or vegetable salads.
- ✦ Use as a binder in croquettes.
- ✦ Use in sauces and gelatin dishes.

GRANOLA
- ✦ Use in cookie, muffin, and bread batters.
- ✦ Sprinkle on vegetables, yogurt, ice cream, pudding, custard, and fruit.
- ✦ Layer with fruits and bake.
- ✦ Mix with dry fruits and nuts for a snack.
- ✦ Substitute for bread or rice in pudding recipes.

DRIED FRUIT
- ✦ Try cooking dried fruits for breakfast, snack or dessert.
- ✦ Add to muffins, cookies, breads, cakes, rice and grain dishes, cereals, puddings, and stuffings.

- ✦ Add to bake in pies and turnovers.
- ✦ Combine with cooked vegetables, such as carrots, sweet potatoes, yams, and acorn squash and butternut squash.
- ✦ Combine with nuts or granola for snacks.

BUTTER OR MARGARINE

- ✦ Add to soups, mashed and baked potatoes, hot cereals, grits, rice, noodles, and cooked vegetables.
- ✦ Stir into cream soups, sauces, and gravies.
- ✦ Combine with herbs and seasonings, and spread on cooked meats, hamburgers, and fish and egg dishes.
- ✦ Use melted butter or margarine as a dip for seafood and raw vegetables, such as shrimp, scallops, crab, and lobster.

Shopping List for High Calorie and High Protein Foods

- ✦ Applesauce
- ✦ Beans, assorted canned
- ✦ Beef
- ✦ Biscuits
- ✦ Bread
- ✦ Butter
- ✦ Cheese
- ✦ Chicken, skinless, boneless
- ✦ Cottage cheese
- ✦ Cereal
- ✦ Cream of wheat
- ✦ Eggs
- ✦ Fish, salmon, tuna, shrimp
- ✦ Fruit, fresh, frozen, canned, dried
- ✦ Grits
- ✦ Honey
- ✦ Ice cream, frozen yogurt
- ✦ Milk, butttermilk, half-and-half
- ✦ Nutritional energy drink supplement
- ✦ Nuts
- ✦ Oatmeal
- ✦ Pasta
- ✦ Peanut Butter
- ✦ Pizza Crust
- ✦ Popsicles
- ✦ Potatoes
- ✦ Pretzels
- ✦ Puddings, flavored gelatins
- ✦ Tomato sauce
- ✦ Tortillas
- ✦ Vegetables, fresh, frozen, canned
- ✦ Whipped topping, frozen
- ✦ Yogurt

Menus

Foods to eat when weight loss is occurring.

Breakfast

153   Tasty Tropical Smoothie
154   Shrimp and Cheese Grits
196   Coffee Cake

Lunch or Dinner

170   Easy Brisket
40   Cheesy Macaroni
239   Squash and Tomato Casserole
259   Strawberry Angel Food Cake

171   Smothered Round Steak
161   Mashed Potatoes
111   Basic Broccoli
49   Chess Pie

160   Quick Black Bean Soup
37   Tuna Salad
80   Easy Banana Bread
198   Mocha Meringue Mounds

Brie and Cranberry Chutney
Quesadillas   156
Easy Beef Enchiladas   164

Caesar Salad   230
Lemon Chicken with Feta   167
Linguine Florentine   62

Pork Medallions   172
Vegetables au Gratin   162
Rice
Cream Cheese Bread Pudding   145

Tropical Green Salad   232
Burger Soup *or* Easy Chili   158 and 159
Yam Biscuits   48
Mock Chocolate Éclair   52

Vegetarian

Sweet Potato Bisque   157
Spinach and Black Bean Enchiladas   163
German Chocolate Angel Pie   144

Any recipes in the book may also be used in this section.

Tasty Tropical Smoothie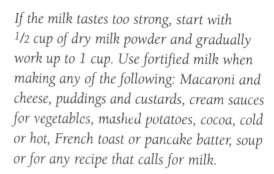

Smoothies are a great snack or meal substitute when you don't have an appetite.

MAKES 1 SERVING

1 ripe banana, sliced
1/2 cup chopped peaches (fresh or frozen)
1 cup mango, papaya, peach nectar or juice
1/2 cup milk (any type) or nutritional energy
  drink supplement
4 ice cubes

Place the banana, peaches, nectar, milk and ice in a blender or food processor. Blend all ingredients together to the desired consistency. Add additional liquid if needed.

Nutrition information per serving
Calories 326, Protein (g) 7, Carbohydrate (g) 79, Fat (g) 1, Calories from Fat (%) 3, Saturated Fat (g) 0, Dietary Fiber (g) 6, Cholesterol (mg) 2, Sodium (mg) 59, Diabetic Exchanges: 5 fruit, 1/2 skim milk

DOC'S NOTES:

In any smoothie recipe, use whichever liquid you prefer: soy milk, rice milk, almond milk, oat milk, regular non-fat milk or liquid nutritional supplements.

Fortified Milk

If the milk tastes too strong, start with 1/2 cup of dry milk powder and gradually work up to 1 cup. Use fortified milk when making any of the following: Macaroni and cheese, puddings and custards, cream sauces for vegetables, mashed potatoes, cocoa, cold or hot, French toast or pancake batter, soup or for any recipe that calls for milk.

MAKES 1 QUART

1 quart whole milk
1 cup nonfat instant dry milk

Pour liquid milk into a deep bowl. Add dry milk and beat slowly with beater until dry milk is dissolved (usually less than five minutes). Refrigerate and serve cold.

Nutrition information per 1 cup serving
Calories 212, Protein (g) 15, Carbohydrate (g) 20, Fat (g) 8, Calories from Fat (%) 34, Saturated Fat (g) 5, Dietary Fiber (g) 0, Cholesterol (mg) 24, Sodium (mg) 200, Diabetic Exchanges: 2 skim milk, 1 1/2 fat

DOC'S NOTES

Milk is a high quality protein and is rich in calcium, vitamins A, D, phosphorus, and magnesium. Milk is the foundation for all other dairy products.

Shrimp and Cheese Grits ❄

This speedy shrimp mixed with cheesy seasoned grits and ham makes a one-meal breakfast. The shrimp may be omitted or adjust the recipe to your tastes.

MAKES 4 TO 6 SERVINGS

1 cup quick grits
3½ cups skim milk
1½ cups shredded reduced-fat sharp Cheddar cheese, divided
¼ cup grated Parmesan cheese
½ teaspoon paprika
Dash of cayenne pepper
⅓ cup diced Canadian bacon
Salt and pepper to taste
1 pound medium peeled shrimp
1 teaspoon minced garlic
1 tablespoon lemon juice
Salt and pepper, to taste
½ cup chopped green onions (scallions)

In a medium pot, cook grits in the milk according to instructions on package. When the grits are ready, stir in Cheddar cheese, the Parmesan cheese, paprika, and cayenne pepper until the cheese is melted. Coat a large nonstick skillet with nonstick cooking spray and cook the bacon, over medium heat, until the bacon begins to brown. Add the shrimp and garlic, cook, stirring, until the shrimp are fully pink and almost done, 3 to 5 minutes. Add the lemon juice, and cook, stirring, until the shrimp are done. Remove from the heat and stir in the grits mixture. Season with salt and pepper. Stir in the green onions. Serve immediately. For later use, milk may need to be added if too thick.

Nutrition information per serving
Calories 309, Protein (g) 30, Carbohydrate (g) 29, Fat (g) 7, Calories from Fat (%) 22, Saturated Fat (g) 5, Dietary Fiber (g) 1, Cholesterol (mg) 137, Sodium (mg) 519, Diabetic Exchanges: 3 lean meat, 1½ starch, ½ skim milk

DOC'S NOTES:

Shrimp are low in fat and calories but higher in cholesterol than most seafood.

Southwestern Egg Wraps 🥕

Here's a fun way to serve scrambled eggs filled with cheese, salsa, and lots of pizzazz. Eggbeaters may be substituted for the eggs.

MAKES 6 TO 8 SERVINGS

3 tablespoons chopped green chilies

1 bunch green onions (scallions), finely chopped

4 eggs

5 egg whites

¼ cup skim milk

1 teaspoon ground cumin

Salt and pepper to taste

6 to 8 (6-inch) flour or corn tortillas, heated in the microwave to soften

2 cups shredded reduced-fat sharp Cheddar cheese or Monterey Jack cheese

In a bowl, mix the green chiles, green onions, eggs, egg whites, milk, cumin, and salt and pepper. Pour the egg mixture into a nonstick skillet coated with nonstick cooking spray over medium heat. Scramble eggs until done. Divide the eggs between the tortillas, sprinkle with cheese and salsa. Roll up and serve immediately.

Nutrition information per serving

Calories 236, Protein (g) 16, Carbohydrate (g) 19, Fat (g) 10, Calories from Fat (%) 38, Saturated Fat (g) 5, Dietary Fiber (g) 2, Cholesterol (mg) 121, Sodium (mg) 418, Diabetic Exchanges: 2 lean meat, 1.5 starch, 0.5 fat

DOC'S NOTES:

The amount of eggs or egg beaters may be used as desired. Breakfast dishes are a good way to get protein in the day.

Brie and Cranberry Chutney Quesadillas 🥕

These quesadillas make a quick meal or snack and a foundation for adding other ingredients. Load them up with a variety of ingredients including leftover meat or chicken for added protein.

MAKES 24 WEDGES

6 (8 to 10-inch) flour tortillas
1 (9-ounce) jar cranberry chutney
8 ounces Brie cheese, rind removed and sliced
2/3 cup chopped chicken breasts, turkey or
   pork tenderloin.

Preheat the oven to 425 degrees. Spread one side of the tortilla with the cranberry chutney and top with sliced Brie. Add whatever meat desired. Fold in half, pressing the edges together. Lay on baking sheet coated with nonstick cooking spray and bake until the cheese is melted and the tortillas are golden. Let sit a few minutes before cutting into wedges.

Nutrition information per serving
Calories 86, Protein (g) 4, Carbohydrate (g) 10, Fat (g) 3, Calories from Fat (%) 33, Saturated Fat (g) 2, Dietary Fiber (g) 1, Cholesterol (mg) 13, Sodium (mg) 153, Diabetic Exchanges: 0.5 lean meat, 0.5 starch

DOC'S NOTES:

Sneak in protein with lean meat in a quick snack. Add veggies for extra nutrition.

HIGH CALORIE
HIGH PROTEIN

Sweet Potato Bisque 🥕 ❄️

This smooth sweet potato soup hits the spot when you want creamed soup.

MAKES 4 CUPS

1 tablespoon butter

1 onion, chopped

3 cups (1/2-inch) chunks peeled sweet potatoes (yam)

2 cups canned chicken or vegetable broth

1/2 teaspoon dried thyme leaves

1/8 teaspoon cayenne

1 cup skim milk

Salt and pepper to taste

In a large non-stick pot, melt the butter and sauté the onion until tender, about 4 minutes. Add the sweet potato and chicken broth and bring to a boil. Reduce the heat and simmer, covered, for 15 minutes, or until the potatoes are tender. Pour the mixture into a food processor and blend until smooth; return to the pot. Add the thyme, cayenne pepper, and milk and cook over a low heat just until heated through. Season to taste.

Nutrition information per serving

Calories 156, Protein (g) 5, Carbohydrate (g) 27, Fat (g) 3, Calories from Fat (%) 18, Saturated Fat (g) 2, Dietary Fiber (g) 4, Cholesterol (mg) 9, Sodium (mg) 296, Diabetic Exchanges: 1.5 starch, 1 vegetable

DOC'S NOTES:

Sweet potatoes provide a great source of beta-carotene and fiber and has been touted as one of the most nutritious vegetables.

Burger Soup ❄

Ground meat anchors this simple veggie soup filled with carrots, corn and rice, giving the soup its name.

MAKES 6 SERVINGS

1 pound ground sirloin
1 onion, chopped
1 teaspoon minced garlic
1 (15-ounce) can tomato sauce
1 (14½-ounce) can chopped tomatoes
4 cups water
Salt and pepper to taste
1 tablespoon Worcestershire sauce
1 bay leaf
1 cup sliced peeled carrots
1½ cups frozen corn
⅓ cup rice

In a large pot, cook the meat, onion, and garlic until the meat is done. Drain excess liquid. Add the tomato sauce, tomatoes, water, salt and pepper, Worcestershire sauce, bay leaf, and carrots. Bring to a boil, reduce heat, and cook for 10 minutes. Add the corn and rice and continue cooking over a medium heat until the rice is done and the carrots are tender, about 30 to 40 minutes. Add more water if too thick.

Nutrition information per serving
Calories 212, Protein (g) 19, Carbohydrate (g) 29, Fat (g) 4, Calories from Fat (%) 15, Saturated Fat (g) 1, Dietary Fiber (g) 3, Cholesterol (mg) 40, Sodium (mg) 590, Diabetic Exchanges: 2 lean meat, 1½ starch, 1½ vegetable

DOC'S NOTES:

Corn, carrots, and tomatoes provide vitamin C, while the tomatoes and carrots are an excellent source of vitamin A.

Easy Chili ❄

Meat, salsa, corn, beef broth and beans are the foundation for this incredible quick favorite chili.

MAKES 6 TO 8 SERVINGS

2 pounds ground sirloin

1 teaspoon minced garlic

1 tablespoon chili powder

1 teaspoon ground cumin

1 (16-ounce) jar chunky salsa

1 (16-ounce) package frozen corn

2 (14½-ounce) cans seasoned beef broth

1 (15-ounce) can pinto beans, drained and rinsed

In a large pot, brown the meat and garlic until the meat is cooked through. Drain any excess liquid. Add the chili powder, cumin, salsa, corn, beef broth, and beans. Bring the mixture to a boil, reduce heat and cook for 15 minutes.

Nutrition information per serving

Calories 266, Protein (g) 29, Carbohydrate (g) 25, Fat (g) 7, Calories from Fat (%) 22, Saturated Fat (g) 2, Dietary Fiber (g) 5, Cholesterol (mg) 60, Sodium (mg) 848, Diabetic Exchanges: 3 lean meat, 1½ starch, 1 vegetable

DOC'S NOTES:

Meat provides protein and iron while the corn and beans are a good source of vitamin C, and folacin.

HIGH CALORIE
HIGH PROTEIN

Quick Black Bean Soup 🥕 ❄️

Cans of black beans and broth turn a black bean soup into a snappy simple soup. Serve with a dollop of fat free sour cream, chopped green onions, and a sprinkle of Cheddar cheese, if desired.

MAKES 8 CUPS

1 onion, chopped
1 green bell pepper, seeded and chopped
1 teaspoon minced garlic
1 (14½-ounce) can chopped tomatoes with juice
1 teaspoon ground cumin
1 teaspoon chili powder
4 (16-ounce) cans black beans, rinsed
  and drained
4 cups chicken or vegetable broth
Salt and pepper to taste

In a large pot coated with nonstick cooking spray, sauté the onion, bell pepper and onion until very tender, about 7 minutes. Mix in tomatoes and juice, cumin and chili powder. Gradually add the black beans and chicken broth. Remove 2 cups of the black bean mixture, and purée in the processor or blender until smooth. Return puréed mixture to pot of soup, bring to a boil, lower heat and simmer for 10 to 15 minutes. Season to taste.

Nutrition information per serving
Calories 222, Protein (g) 14, Carbohydrate (g) 35, Fat (g) 2, Calories from Fat (%) 8, Saturated Fat (g) 0, Dietary Fiber (g) 13, Cholesterol (mg) 0, Sodium (mg) 981, Diabetic Exchanges: 1 very lean meat, 2 starch, 1 vegetable

HIGH CALORIE
HIGH PROTEIN

DOC'S NOTES:

Beans sneak in protein and fiber when you are looking for a meatless choice. Use reduced sodium chicken broth to reduce sodium in recipe.

Mashed Potatoes

Nothing beats the comfort food of plain mashed potatoes.

MAKES 6 TO 8 SERVINGS

2 1/2 pounds baking potatoes, peeled
  and quartered
3 tablespoons margarine
2/3 cup skim milk, warmed
1/3 cup plain nonfat yogurt
Salt and pepper to taste
1/2 cup chopped green onions (scallions)

Combine the potatoes and enough water to cover in a large nonstick saucepan; bring to a boil. Lower the heat, cover, and cook until tender about 20 to 25 minutes; drain. In a bowl, mash the potatoes with the margarine, milk and yogurt until creamy. Season to taste. Transfer to serving dish, sprinkle with green onions and serve.

Nutrition information per serving

Calories 159, Protein (g) 4, Carbohydrate (g) 27, Fat (g) 4, Calories from Fat (%) 25, Saturated Fat (g) 1, Dietary Fiber (g) 2, Cholesterol (mg) 1, Sodium (mg) 74, Diabetic Exchanges: 2 starch, 0.5 fat

DOC'S NOTES:

Easy on the stomach, and potatoes are filled with vitamins B6, C, iron, magnesium and niacin. Niacin helps in the conversion or food into energy. It helps to maintain normal functions of the skin, nerves, and digestive system.

Vegetable au Gratin 🥕

Veggies smothered with a white sauce and cheese makes a vegetarian entrée or an outstanding side.

MAKES 4 TO 6 SERVINGS

4 large red potatoes (about 1½ pounds), sliced
¾ pound fresh green beans, ends snapped
1 pound yellow squash, sliced
Salt and pepper to taste
2 cups shredded reduced fat sharp Cheddar cheese, divided
1 cup frozen green peas, thawed
2 cups skim milk
⅓ cup all-purpose flour

Preheat the oven to 350 degrees. Cook potatoes, green beans, and squash in a little water in microwave or on stove until crisp tender. Spread the potatoes in the bottom of a 2-quart oblong casserole coated with nonstick cooking spray and sprinkle with salt and pepper and 1 cup cheese. Top with green beans. Layer squash and peas on top. In a small pot, combine the milk and flour, stirring, over a medium heat until thickened. Pour evenly over the top of layered veggies. Sprinkle with remaining 1 cup cheese. Bake for 20 minutes or until heated through.

Nutrition information per serving

Calories 297, Protein (g) 20, Carbohydrate (g) 40, Fat (g) 7, Calories from Fat (%) 21, Saturated Fat (g) 5, Dietary Fiber (g) 5, Cholesterol (mg) 22, Sodium (mg) 312, Diabetic Exchanges: 2 lean meat, 2 starch, 2 vegetable

DOC'S NOTES:

Beans, peas and squash are filled with vitamins A, C, and folacin. Potatoes are rich in vitamins B6, C, iron, magnesium and niacin.

HIGH CALORIE
HIGH PROTEIN

Spinach and Black Bean Enchiladas

These simple ingredients give "tons of flavor" to this meatless enchilada, making it a quick and favorite standby. To reduce sodium, substitute 1 teaspoon each chili powder and ground cumin for taco seasoning mix

MAKES 8 ENCHILADAS

1 (10-ounce) package frozen spinach, thawed
1 (15-ounce) can black beans, rinsed and drained
1 (1.25 ounce) package low sodium taco seasoning mix
1 cup water
1 cup nonfat sour cream, divided
1 (10-ounce) can enchilada sauce
8 (6 to 8-inch) tortillas
1 cup shredded reduced fat Cheddar cheese
2 tablespoons chopped green onions (scallions)

Preheat 375 degrees. In a skillet coated with nonstick cooking spray, heat the spinach, black beans, taco seasoning mix, and water. Bring to a boil, reduce heat, and cook for 8 to 10 minutes or until mixture is thickened. Remove from heat and stir in $1/2$ cup sour cream. On each tortilla, spread 1 tablespoon enchilada sauce, about $1/3$ cup spinach mixture, and one heaping tablespoon cheese. Roll up each tortilla placing seam side down in an oblong baking dish coated with nonstick cooking spray. Spread remaining enchilada sauce over filled enchiladas, cover, and bake 15 to 18 minutes. Serve with remaining sour cream and sprinkle with green onions.

Nutrition information per serving
Calories 238, Protein (g) 13, Carbohydrate (g) 38, Fat (g) 3, Calories from Fat (%) 13, Saturated Fat (g) 2, Dietary Fiber (g) 5, Cholesterol (mg) 13, Sodium (mg) 969, Diabetic Exchanges: 1 lean meat, 2.5 starch

DOC'S NOTES:

Black beans provide protein, iron and calcium while spinach is packed with vitamins A, C, folacin, iron and magnesium.

Easy Beef Enchiladas ❄

Hard to believe this effortless recipe makes such an outstanding enchilada. For increased calories, use regular products instead of nonfat and load on the cheese for extra protein. Add black beans or pinto beans for my favorite version and added protein.

MAKES 10 TO 12 ENCHILADAS

1¼ pounds ground sirloin
1 onion, chopped
Salt and pepper to taste
1 cup nonfat sour cream
1 cup frozen corn
2 cups canned mild enchilada sauce, divided
2 cups reduced fat Mexican blend, Monterey Jack
  or Cheddar cheese, divided
10 to 12 (6 to 8-inch) tortillas

Preheat the oven to 350 degrees. In a large skillet, cook the meat and onion over medium heat for about 6 to 8 minutes or until meat is done. Drain any excess grease. Remove from heat and stir in the sour cream, corn, and ¼ cup enchilada sauce. Spread about ⅓ cup enchilada sauce on the bottom of a 13×9×2-inch baking dish coated with nonstick cooking spray. Spoon about 2 tablespoons meat mixture and about 1 tablespoon cheese onto each tortilla. Roll tortilla around filling and place seam side down on sauce in baking dish. Pour remaining sauce over the filled enchiladas. Sprinkle with remaining cheese. Bake for 15 to 18 minutes or until cheese melted and enchiladas heated.

Nutrition information per serving
Calories 197, Protein (g) 11, Carbohydrate (g) 29, Fat (g) 4, Calories from Fat (%) 18, Saturated Fat (g) 3, Dietary Fiber (g) 2, Cholesterol (mg) 15, Sodium (mg) 591, Diabetic Exchanges: 1 lean meat, 2 starch

DOC'S NOTES:

Corn provides fiber and complex carbohydrates. It is also a good source of folacin, magnesium and phosphorous.

HIGH CALORIE
HIGH PROTEIN

Quick Loaded Chicken Enchiladas ❄

Save a step and purchase Rotessire chicken to toss in with the salsa. Follow remaining directions to create this outstanding simple enchilada recipe filled with salsa, touch of cumin and cheese.

MAKES 6 SERVINGS

3 slices center-cut bacon, cut in pieces
1¼ pounds skinless boneless chicken breasts, cut in cubes
½ teaspoon minced garlic
1½ cups salsa, divided
1 (15-ounce) can black beans, drained and rinsed
1 red bell pepper, seeded and chopped, optional
1 teaspoon ground cumin
Salt and pepper to taste
1 bunch green onions (scallions), chopped
12 (6- to 8-inch) flour tortillas
1½ cups shredded reduced fat Monterey Jack or Mexican blend cheese

Preheat oven to 350 degrees. In a skillet, cook bacon until crisp. Remove bacon to paper towel to soak any excess grease and discard any grease in skillet. In the same skillet coated with nonstick cooking spray, sauté chicken and garlic until chicken is almost done. Stir in ½ cup salsa, beans, bell pepper, cumin, and salt and pepper to taste. Simmer about 5 minutes, stirring occasionally until chicken is done. Stir in green onions and reserved bacon. Divide chicken bean mixture among 12 tortillas, sprinkle with about 1 tablespoon cheese and roll up placing seam side down in 13×9×2-inch baking dish coated with nonstick cooking spray. Spoon remaining 1 cup salsa evenly over enchiladas and sprinkle with remaining cheese. Bake for 15 minutes or until thoroughly heated and cheese is melted.

Nutrition information per serving

Calories 464, Protein (g) 39, Carbohydrate (g) 53, Fat (g) 8, Calories from Fat (%) 16, Saturated Fat (g) 4, Dietary Fiber (g) 7, Cholesterol (mg) 73, Sodium (mg) 1282, Diabetic Exchanges: 4 lean meat, 3 starch, 1.5 vegetable

DOC'S NOTES:

Chicken provides protein, vitamins B6, B12 and niacin and phosphorus.

Ginger Chicken and Black Beans ❄

Peaches, ginger, and black beans join together for this wonderful sweet and savory dish.

MAKES 6 SERVINGS

2½ pounds skinless, boneless chicken breasts

Salt and pepper to taste

½ teaspoon garlic powder

1 teaspoon paprika

1 (15-ounce) can light sliced peaches, drained and cut into chunks

1 teaspoon ground ginger

2 tablespoons lime juice

1 teaspoon minced garlic

½ cup chopped green onions (scallions)

2 (15-ounce) cans black beans, undrained

Preheat oven to 350 degrees. Place the chicken in a 2-quart oblong baking dish. Season with the salt and pepper, garlic powder, and paprika. In a bowl, combine the peaches, ginger, lime juice, garlic, green onions, and black beans. Spoon this mixture over the chicken, cover, and bake for 45 to 60 minutes, or until the chicken is tender.

Nutrition information per serving

Calories 363, Protein (g) 51, Carbohydrate (g) 27, Fat (g) 4, Calories from Fat (%) 9, Saturated Fat (g) 1, Dietary Fiber (g) 9, Cholesterol (mg) 110, Sodium (mg) 567, Diabetic Exchanges: 6 very lean meat, 1.5 starch, 0.5 fruit

DOC'S NOTES:

This recipe is high in calories and high in protein with a palate-pleasing flavor. Ginger is supposed to be soothing to your stomach.

HIGH CALORIE
HIGH PROTEIN

Lemon Chicken
with Feta ❄

Four ingredients cooked with chicken create an instant dinner success. The lemon flavor might help with cancer patients.

MAKES 8 SERVINGS

8 skinless, boneless chicken breasts
1/4 cup lemon juice, divided
1 tablespoon dried oregano leaves, divided
Salt and pepper to taste
4 ounces crumbled feta cheese
3 tablespoons chopped green onions (scallions)

Preheat oven to 350 degrees. Place the chicken in a 13×9×2-inch baking dish coated with nonstick cooking spray and drizzle with half of the lemon juice. Sprinkle with half of the oregano and salt and pepper. Sprinkle with the cheese and green onions. Drizzle with the remaining lemon juice and oregano. Bake, covered, for 45 minutes to 1 hour, or until done.

Nutrition information per serving
Calories 172, Protein (g) 29, Carbohydrate (g) 2, Fat (g) 5, Calories from Fat (%) 25, Saturated Fat (g) 3, Dietary Fiber (g) 0, Cholesterol (mg) 81, Sodium (mg) 236, Diabetic Exchanges: 4 very lean meat

DOC'S NOTES:

Chicken provides protein as well as vitamin B6, B12, niacin and phosphorus. Vitamin B12 is important for metabolism. It aids in red blood cell formation and helps maintain the central nervous system.

Shrimp Scampi with White Beans ❄

A trouble-free and quick scampi recipe with asparagus and white beans tossed with fettuccine makes an instant one-meal dish. Chicken may be substituted for the shrimp. If using chicken, cook the chicken first in the skillet in the oil and proceed with recipe adding asparagus.

MAKES 4 SERVINGS

2 tablespoons olive oil

1 pound asparagus, cut into 1 inch pieces

1 tablespoon minced garlic

1 pound medium shrimp, peeled

1½ cups coarsely chopped Roma tomatoes

1 (16-ounce) can Great Northern beans, or navy beans, rinsed and drained

1 cup low sodium chicken broth

2 teaspoon cornstarch

½ teaspoon dried basil leaves

Salt and pepper to taste

½ pound spinach fettuccine, cooked according to package directions

2 tablespoons grated Parmesan cheese

In a large nonstick skillet, heat the oil over medium heat and cook the asparagus and garlic for 1 to 2 minutes, stirring. Add shrimp and cook until pink, about 3 minutes. Add the tomatoes and beans, cooking for another 3 minutes or until tomatoes are softened. In a small bowl, mix together the chicken broth and cornstarch, stir into skillet. Cook over medium heat until thickened, stirring frequently. Add basil and season to taste. Serve over fettuccine and sprinkle with cheese.

Nutrition information per serving

Calories 486, Protein (g) 34, Carbohydrate (g) 65, Fat (g) 10, Calories from Fat (%) 19, Saturated Fat (g) 2, Dietary Fiber (g) 12, Cholesterol (mg) 149, Sodium (mg) 676, Diabetic Exchanges: 3 lean meat, 4 starch, 1 vegetable

DOC'S NOTES:

Asparagus provides a great source of vitamins A, B6, C, E, an folacin. Beans provide fiber, iron, and vitamin C.

HIGH CALORIE
HIGH PROTEIN

Indoor Barbecue
Roasted Salmon ❄

Simple seasonings perk up the salmon with a sweet spicy rub. Easy to make and enjoyable to eat.

MAKES 4 SERVINGS

4 (6-ounce) salmon fillets
2 tablespoons light brown sugar
4 teaspoons chili powder
1 teaspoon ground cumin
1/4 teaspoon ground cinnamon
Salt and pepper to taste

Preheat oven to 400° F. In a small bowl, mix together the brown sugar, chili powder, cumin, cinnamon and salt and pepper. Rub over the salmon and place in an 11×7×2-inch baking dish coated with nonstick cooking spray. Bake for 12 to 15 minutes or until fish flakes easily when tested with a fork.

Nutrition information per serving
Calories 234, Protein (g) 34, Carbohydrate (g) 8, Fat (g) 6, Calories from Fat (%) 25, Saturated Fat (g) 1, Dietary Fiber (g) 1, Cholesterol (mg) 88, Sodium (mg) 144, Diabetic Exchanges: 5 very lean meat, 0.5 other carbohydrate

DOC'S NOTES:

Salmon is a good source of Vitamin B12, niacin, phosphorus and a great source of those heart-healthy omega 3s.

Easy Brisket ❄

This is one of my old standby simple-to-prepare recipes I have made for years and continually go back to. Pop the brisket in the oven, forget about the brisket, and the end result is this succulent tender brisket, and leftovers make incredible sandwiches. This recipe can be made in the slow cooker.

MAKES 12 TO 14 SERVINGS

5 to 6 pound very lean brisket, trimmed of
  excess fat
Garlic powder
1 cup light brown sugar
1 cup water
1 envelope dry onion soup mix
1 cup ketchup

Preheat the oven to 325° F. Season the brisket heavily with the garlic powder. In a small bowl, mix together the brown sugar, water, onion soup mix, and ketchup. Pour over the brisket in a large baking pan or roaster. Cook, covered, for 4 1/2 hours to 5 hours or hours, or until meat is fork tender. To serve, slice against the grain and serve with sauce.

Nutrition information per serving
Calories 330, Protein (g) 40, Carbohydrate (g) 21, Fat (g) 9, Calories from Fat (%) 24, Saturated Fat (g) 3, Dietary Fiber (g) 0, Cholesterol (mg) 83, Sodium (mg) 435, Diabetic Exchanges: 5 1/2 lean meat, 1 1/2 other carbohydrate

DOC'S NOTES:

The lean brisket is a good source of iron, zinc and vitamins B6 and B12.

Smothered Round Steak ❄

Round steak cooked in incredible brown seasoned gravy is great served over mashed potatoes, pasta or rice. This lean cut of meat needs a longer cooking time to tenderize; but it is worth the wait.

MAKES 6 SERVINGS

3 pounds lean, boneless top round steak, trimmed of excess fat

1/4 teaspoon pepper

1/4 cup all-purpose flour

1 onion, thickly sliced

2 green bell peppers, seeded and sliced

1 tablespoon minced garlic

2 cups canned beef broth

1 (15-ounce) can tomato sauce

1 teaspoon light brown sugar

1 tablespoon Worcestershire sauce

1 teaspoon dried basil leaves

1 teaspoon dried thyme leaves

1 teaspoon dried oregano leaves

Season the steak with the pepper and coat in the flour, shaking off any excess. In a large nonstick skillet coated with nonstick cooking spray, brown the steak over medium heat for 5 to 7 minutes on each side. Remove the steak and set aside. Add the onion and bell pepper to the skillet and cook over moderate heat, stirring occasionally, about 5 minutes. Stir in the garlic, beef broth, tomato sauce, brown sugar, Worcestershire sauce, basil, thyme, and oregano and bring to a boil. Return the steak to the skillet. Cover and cook over medium-low heat for 1 1/2 to 2 hours, or until the steak is very tender, stirring occasionally.

Nutrition information per serving
Calories 353, Protein (g) 55, Carbohydrate (g) 14, Fat (g) 8, Calories from Fat (%) 20, Saturated Fat (g) 2, Dietary Fiber (g) 2, Cholesterol (mg) 127, Sodium (mg) 806, Diabetic Exchanges: 7 very lean meat, 3 vegetable

DOC'S NOTES:

You do not need to eat meat to survive, but meat provides iron, zinc, and vitamins B6- and B12-nutrients that are difficult to obtain in a meatless diet.

Pork Medallions ❄

Theses these mouth-watering pork tenderloin medallions cooked with a lemon butter sauce are easy to make. Serve with rice, pasta or potatoes.

MAKES 6 TO 8 SERVINGS

2 pounds pork tenderloin, cut crosswise into
  16 slices, each about 1-inch thick
Salt and pepper to taste
3 tablespoons margarine
¼ cup lemon juice
2 tablespoons Worcestershire sauce
1 tablespoon Dijon mustard
1 tablespoon chopped parsley

Season the pork slices with salt and pepper. Heat the margarine in a nonstick skillet and cook the slices 3 to 4 minutes on each side until browned, working in batches if necessary. Remove to a serving platter and cover to keep warm. Add the lemon juice, Worcestershire sauce, and mustard to the same skillet. Cook, stirring with the pork juices, until heated thoroughly. Return the pork to the sauce, cooking until well heated and done. Sprinkle with parsley and serve.

Nutrition information per serving
Calories 177, Protein (g) 23, Carbohydrate (g) 2, Fat (g) 8, Calories from Fat (%) 43, Saturated Fat (g) 2, Dietary Fiber (g) 0, Cholesterol (mg) 63, Sodium (mg) 175, Diabetic Exchanges: 3 lean meat

DOC'S NOTES:

Meat provides iron, zinc and vitamins B6 and B12. B6, like B12, aids in the formation of red blood cells and helps maintain normal brain function.

HIGH CALORIE
HIGH PROTEIN

Veal and Broccoli with Tomato Vinaigrette ✳

For a nice change, try this light veal dish with a sensational vinaigrette. Serve with pasta.

MAKES 6 SERVINGS

2 cups broccoli florets
1½ pounds thinly sliced veal (scaloppini)
Salt and pepper to taste
¼ cup all-purpose flour
2 tablespoons olive oil
½ cup chopped green onions (scallions)
1½ cups fat free chicken broth
2 teaspoons cornstarch
1 tablespoon water
1 tablespoon balsamic vinegar
1 teaspoon Dijon mustard
2 cups chopped Roma (plum) tomatoes

In a microwave-proof dish, cook the broccoli in ½ cup water until tender-crisp, about 5 to 7 minutes. Drain water, set aside. Season veal with salt and pepper and then dust with flour.

In a large nonstick skillet coated with nonstick cooking spray, heat the olive oil over a medium heat and cook the veal about 3 minutes on each side, until lightly browned. Add the green onions and chicken broth.

In a small cup, blend together the cornstarch and water; add to the pan, stirring until mixture comes to a boil. Reduce heat, cooking until thickened. Stir in the vinegar, mustard, tomatoes and broccoli; cook until heated through, about 3 minutes.

Nutrition information per serving
Calories 218, Protein (g) 25, Carbohydrate (g) 10, Fat (g) 8, Calories from Fat (%) 34, Saturated Fat (g) 2, Dietary Fiber (g) 2, Cholesterol (mg) 94, Sodium (mg) 225, Diabetic Exchanges: 3 lean meat, 2 vegetable

DOC'S NOTES:

Broccoli is in the cruciferous family known for cancer-fighting antioxidants and tomatoes are packed with lycopene.

Ziti with Broccoli and White Beans Topped with Tuna

Slices of tuna top pasta tossed with broccoli and white beans in a light broth sauce. Seasoning the tuna with salt and pepper and searing is simple and delicious. The tuna may be omitted for a pasta-only dish.

MAKES 4 TO 6 SERVINGS

12 ounces ziti pasta

2 tablespoons olive oil

4 cups broccoli florets

1 teaspoon minced garlic

1/2 cup white wine

1/2 cup chicken broth

1 (16-ounce) can cannelloni beans, drained and rinsed

1/4 cup grated Parmesan cheese

16 ounces tuna fillets

Salt and pepper taste

Prepare pasta according to package directions. Drain and set aside. In a large nonstick skillet, heat the olive oil over medium heat and stir-fry the broccoli and garlic until the broccoli is tender. Add the wine, chicken broth and cannelloni beans. Bring to a boil; reduce heat and cook about 5 to 7 minutes longer. Add pasta and toss together. Meanwhile, season tuna with salt and pepper. Heat a nonstick skillet with nonstick cooking spray and sear the tuna on both sides, about 3 minutes. Do not overcook. Slice the tuna and serve over the pasta dish.

Nutrition information per serving
Calories 429, Protein (g) 30, Carbohydrate (g) 56, Fat (g) 8, Calories from Fat (%) 16, Saturated Fat (g) 2, Dietary Fiber (g) 6, Cholesterol (mg) 38, Sodium (mg) 261, Diabetic Exchanges: 3 lean meat, 3 1/2 starch

DOC'S NOTES:

Tuna is a great source of protein and omega 3 fatty acids, and the beans and cheese are added protein.

Cereal Clusters

These no bake cookies are made with high fiber cereal, peanuts, peanut butter and butterscotch chips are about the best thing you have ever popped in your mouth. These easy addictive clusters make a great pick up any time of day.

MAKES 60 CLUSTERS

1/2 cup peanut butter
1 (11-ounce) bag butterscotch chips
8 cups lightly sweetened whole grain flakes with honey clusters or any lightly sweetened fiber flake cereal with clusters
1 cup coarsely chopped peanuts

In a microwave-safe dish, melt peanut butter and butterscotch chips for 1 to 2 minutes, stirring after 1 minute until melted. In a large bowl, combine the cereal and peanuts and pour the butterscotch mixture over, mixing carefully until the cereal is well coated. Drop by tablespoonfuls on baking sheet lined with wax paper. Refrigerate until firm. When firm, transfer to zip top bags and store in the refrigerator.

Nutrition information per serving
Calories 83, Protein (g) 2, Carbohydrate (g) 10, Fat (g) 4, Calories from Fat (%) 43, Saturated Fat (g) 2, Dietary Fiber (g) 1, Cholesterol (mg) 0, Sodium (mg) 49, Diabetic Exchanges: 1/2 other carbohydrate, 1 fat

DOC'S NOTES:

The whole grain flakes and peanuts provide fiber while the peanuts provide more protein than any other nut. Peanuts are also a good source of iron and magnesium.

HIGH CALORIE
HIGH PROTEIN

Peanut Butter Snack Spread 🥕

A quick and tasty spread to keep around for bagels, crackers, bananas or use as desired. This spread is also good enough to eat with a spoon.

MAKES ½ CUP SPREAD

1 tablespoon nonfat instant dry milk
1 tablespoon water
1 teaspoon vanilla extract
1 tablespoon honey
⅓ cup smooth peanut butter

In a small bowl, combine the dry milk, water, and vanilla, stirring to moisten. Add honey and peanut butter, stirring slowly until blended. Use as spread on crackers. Refrigerate, but if too stiff to spread let sit to room temperature to soften.

Nutrition information per serving
Calories 150, Protein (g) 6, Carbohydrate (g) 10, Fat (g) 11, Calories from Fat (%) 60, Saturated Fat (g) 2, Dietary Fiber (g) 1, Cholesterol (mg) 0, Sodium (mg) 107, Diabetic Exchanges: 1 very lean meat, ½ other carbohydrate, 2 fat

DOC'S NOTES:

The peanuts are high in fiber and protein. Peanuts are also a good source of niacin and folacin.

Fabulous Fruit Dip

Make up this heavenly dip and refrigerate to pull out with fresh fruit as a quick snack. Here's your opportunity to include lots of fruit and lots of dip.

MAKES SIXTEEN (2-TABLESPOON) SERVINGS

1 (7-ounce) jar marshmallow creme
1 (8-ounce) package reduced-fat cream cheese
1 tablespoon grated orange rind
2 tablespoons orange juice

In a mixing bowl, beat together the marshmallow creme and cream cheese until smooth. Stir in the orange rind and orange juice. Refrigerate until ready to serve.

Nutrition information per serving
Calories 78, Protein (g) 2, Carbohydrate (g) 11, Fat (g) 3, Calories from Fat (%) 36, Saturated Fat (g) 2, Dietary Fiber (g) 0, Cholesterol (mg) 10, Sodium (mg) 68, Diabetic Exchanges: 1/2 other carbohydrate, 1/2 fat

DOC'S NOTES:

The cream cheese provides vitamin B12, phosphorus, and calcium. Phosphorus is vital for energy production and in building bones and teeth. A good dip to encourage you to eat more fresh fruit.

HIGH CALORIE
HIGH PROTEIN

Banana Split Dessert 🥕

This scrumptious banana split layered dessert includes all the makings of a sundae with a make ahead plan. Sugar free pudding may be used.

MAKES 12 TO 16 SERVINGS

2 cups graham cracker crumbs
   (about 32 squares)
6 tablespoons margarine, melted
1 (12-ounce) can cold evaporated fat free milk
1/4 cup cold skim milk
2 (4-serving) packages instant vanilla pudding
   and pie filling mix
2 medium firm bananas, sliced
1 (20-ounce) can unsweetened crushed
   pineapple, drained
1 (8-ounce) container fat free frozen whipped
   topping, thawed
1/4 cup chopped walnuts
4 tablespoons chocolate syrup
5 maraschino cherries, quartered

Preheat oven to 375 degrees. Combine cracker crumbs and margarine and press onto the bottom of a 13×9×2-inch baking dish coated with nonstick cooking spray. Bake for 7 to 10 minutes or until browned. Cool completely. In a bowl, whisk the evaporated milk, milk and pudding mixes for 2 minutes or until slightly thickened. Spread pudding evenly over crust. Layer with bananas, pineapple, and whipped topping. Sprinkle with nuts; drizzle with chocolate syrup. Top with cherries. Refrigerate for at least one hour before cutting.

Nutrition information per serving

Calories 228, Protein (g) 3, Carbohydrate (g) 38, Fat (g) 7, Calories from Fat (%) 27, Saturated Fat (g) 1, Dietary Fiber (g) 1, Cholesterol (mg) 1, Sodium (mg) 332, Diabetic Exchanges: 2 starch, 1/2 fruit, 1 fat

DOC'S NOTES:

Pineapple and bananas provide vitamin C while the bananas are a good source of potassium and B6.

HIGH CALORIE
HIGH PROTEIN

Snacks and Light Meals

- Is snacking permissible?
- Should I make snacks ahead of time?

Snacking is not only permissible but strongly encouraged. It is sometimes very hard to sit down for a full five-course meal, but easier to sit down to a thirty minute meal with two to three snacks in between. High calorie, low volume snacks are important to help you to maintain your weight. We will try to offer suggestions for snacks that can be made easily and with minimal effort.

Snack Foods

- Applesauce
- Bread, muffins, and crackers
- Buttered popcorn
- Cakes and cookies made with whole grains, fruits, nuts, wheat germ, or granola
- Cereal
- Cheese (hard or semisoft)
- Cheesecake
- Chocolate milk
- Crackers
- Cream soups
- Dips made with cheese, beans, or sour cream
- Fruit (fresh, canned, dried)
- Gelatin salads and desserts
- Granola
- Hard-boiled and deviled eggs
- Ice cream frozen yogurt, popsicles
- Juices
- Milkshakes, instant breakfast drinks
- Nuts
- Peanut butter
- Pita bread and hummus
- Pizza
- Puddings and custards
- Sandwiches
- Vegetables (raw or cooked)
- Whole or 2% milk
- Yogurt

Snack Recipes

- Snack Mix
- Granola
- Cereal Mixture
- Cereal Clusters
- No Bake Cookies
- Oatmeal Chocolate Cake
- Spinach Dip
- Fresh Fruit Dip
- Fabulous Fruit Dip

Shopping List for Snacks and Light Meals

- ◆ Applesauce
- ◆ Biscuits
- ◆ Bread
- ◆ Butter
- ◆ Cheese
- ◆ Cottage cheese
- ◆ Cereal
- ◆ Cream of wheat
- ◆ Eggs
- ◆ Fruit, fresh, frozen, canned, dried
- ◆ Grits
- ◆ Ice cream, frozen yogurt
- ◆ Honey
- ◆ Milk
- ◆ Nutritional energy drink supplement
- ◆ Nuts
- ◆ Oatmeal
- ◆ Pasta
- ◆ Peanut Butter
- ◆ Pizza Crust
- ◆ Popsicles
- ◆ Potatoes
- ◆ Pretzels
- ◆ Puddings, flavored gelatins
- ◆ Tomato sauce
- ◆ Tortillas
- ◆ Vegetables, fresh, frozen, canned
- ◆ Whipped topping, frozen
- ◆ Yogurt

Strawberry Slush 🥕

Absolutely yummy! You will repeat this recipe often as it is so soothing to drink.

MAKES 1 SERVING

1 cup fresh strawberries, hulled and halved
2 tablespoons sugar
1/2 cup orange juice
1 tablespoon lemon juice

Combine all ingredients in a blender or food processor and process until smooth.

Nutritional information per serving
Calories 202, Protein (g) 2, Carbohydrate (g) 50, Fat (g) 1, Cal. from Fat (%) 3, Saturated Fat (g) 0, Dietary Fiber (g) 4, Cholesterol (mg) 0, Sodium (mg) 3, Diabetic Exchanges: 2 fruit, 1.5 other carb.

DOC'S NOTES:

Get your extra potassium and Vitamin C from these strawberries. If white blood cell count is low, don't use raw fruit.

Cereal Mixture 🥕

Double this recipe and store in a jar. Great snack for everyone.

MAKES SIX (1/2-CUP) SERVINGS

3 tablespoons honey
3 tablespoon margarine
3 tablespoons reduced-fat peanut butter
3 cups cereal (assorted shredded wheat, corn bran chex)

Preheat oven to 175 degrees. In the microwave, combine honey, margarine, and peanut butter and heat until smooth. Toss with cereal, coating well. Spread on a baking sheet and bake for 1 1/2 hours.

Nutritional information per serving
Calories 201, Protein (g) 5, Carbohydrate (g) 30, Fat (g) 9, Cal. from Fat (%) 37, Saturated Fat (g) 2, Dietary Fiber (g) 4, Cholesterol (mg) 0, Sodium (mg) 199, Diabetic Exchanges: 1.5 starch, 0.5 other carb., 1.5 fat

DOC'S NOTES:

Keep this on hand for daily snacking. Every calorie counts. Peanut butter adds protein and the cereal adds fiber, vitamins, and minerals.

SNACKS AND LIGHT MEALS

Snack Mix 🥕

Here's an easy recipe that makes a great snack mix any time of day. Sweet and salty mixes are always a great combo and this mix is addicting!

MAKES TWENTY (1/2-CUP) SERVINGS

3 tablespoons sesame oil
3 tablespoons honey
1 tablespoon soy sauce
1/2 teaspoon garlic salt
1/2 teaspoon onion powder
4 cups crispy wheat cereal squares
6 cups mini pretzels
1 cup soy nuts
1 cup dry roasted peanuts
1 cup candy-coated chocolate pieces

Preheat oven to 250 degrees. Whisk together sesame oil, honey, soy sauce, garlic salt, and onion powder. Toss together cereal squares, pretzels, soy nuts, and peanuts in a large bowl. Drizzle oil mixture over cereal mixture, tossing gently to coat. Scatter mixture on a foil-lined jelly roll pan and bake for 25 minutes, stirring often to prevent too much browning. Turn off oven and let cereal stay in oven for 1 hour to continue crisping. When cool, toss with the chocolate candies. Store in an airtight container for up to one week.

Nutritional information per serving
Calories 242, Protein (g) 8, Carbohydrate (g) 32, Fat (g) 10, Cal. from Fat (%) 37, Saturated Fat (g) 3, Dietary Fiber (g) 3, Cholesterol (mg) 2, Sodium (mg) 400, Diabetic Exchanges: 0.5 very lean meat, 1 starch, 1 other carb., 2 fat

DOC'S NOTES:

Good source of calories and eating this snack will encourage one to drink fluids.

Cinnamon Quick Bread 🥕 ❄️

A quick bread that will appeal at all times as it's not too rich but very tasty.

MAKES 16 SERVINGS

2 cups all-purpose flour
1 teaspoon baking powder
1 teaspoon baking soda
1/2 cup margarine
1 cup plus 1 tablespoon sugar, divided
2 large eggs
1 teaspoon vanilla extract
1 cup buttermilk
1 1/2 teaspoons ground cinnamon

Preheat oven to 350 degrees. In bowl combine flour, baking powder, and baking soda; set aside. In another mixing bowl, blend margarine and 1 cup sugar. Gradually add eggs and vanilla. Stir in flour mixture and buttermilk alternately, mixing until smooth. Transfer half the batter into a 9×5×3-inch loaf pan coated with nonstick cooking spray. In another small bowl mix together remaining 1 tablespoon sugar and cinnamon. Sprinkle a light dusting over the batter. Swirl the cinnamon sugar into the layer of batter with a knife. Cover with remaining batter and cinnamon sugar.

For a crusted effect, don't swirl the top mixture, lightly dust it over the batter. Bake for 50 to 60 minutes or until a toothpick inserted comes out clean.

Nutritional information per serving
Calories 176, Protein (g) 3, Carbohydrate (g) 20, Fat (g) 7, Cal. from Fat (%) 33, Saturated Fat (g) 1, Dietary Fiber (g) 1, Cholesterol (mg) 27, Sodium (mg) 200, Diabetic Exchanges: 1 starch, 0.5 other carb., 1 fat

DOC'S NOTES:

Good snacking food to increase your daily calorie consumption.

SNACKS AND LIGHT MEALS

Spinach Dip

Whichever way you eat this wonderful dip, it will be with a smile. Spread on French bread halves and bake in the oven for wonderful Spinach Bread. Makes a great side veggie dish, also.

MAKES TWELVE (1/4-CUP) SERVINGS

2 (10-ounce) packages frozen chopped spinach
1/2 cup chopped onion
2 tablespoons all-purpose flour
1 (12-ounce) can evaporated skimmed milk
Salt and pepper to taste
1/2 teaspoon garlic powder
1 cup shredded part-skim mozzarella cheese

Preheat oven to 350 degrees. Prepare spinach according to the package directions; drain well. In a small saucepan coated with nonstick cooking spray, sauté the onion over medium heat 5 minutes or until tender. Add the cooked spinach and flour. Gradually stir in milk, salt, pepper, and garlic powder. Cook over medium-high heat until thickened and bubbly. Remove from the heat. Add the mozzarella cheese, stirring just until mixed.

Nutritional information per serving

Calories 68, Protein (g) 6, Carbohydrate (g) 7, Fat (g) 2, Cal. from Fat (%) 22, Saturated Fat (g) 1, Dietary Fiber (g) 2, Cholesterol (mg) 7, Sodium (mg) 116, Diabetic Exchanges: 0.5 lean meat, 0.5 skim milk

DOC'S NOTES:

This is a great source of potassium.

Strawberry Fruit Dip 🥕

Also makes a sensational soup or smoothie.

MAKES 40 (1-TABLESPOON) SERVINGS

1 quart strawberries, stemmed and
  finely chopped
1/4 cup light brown sugar
1/4 cup orange juice
1 cup nonfat vanilla yogurt
1/2 teaspoon grated orange rind

In a bowl, mix all ingredients. Cover and refrigerate.

Nutritional information per serving

Calories 16, Protein (g) 0, Carbohydrate (g) 4, Fat (g) 0, Cal. from Fat (%) 0, Saturated Fat (g) 0, Dietary Fiber (g) 0, Cholesterol (mg) 0, Sodium (mg) 5, Diabetic Exchanges: Free

DOC'S NOTES:

High in Vitamin C. Avoid fresh fruit if low white blood cell count.

Fresh Fruit Dip 🥕

Great dip and nothing could be faster.

MAKES EIGHT (1/4-CUP) SERVINGS

2 (8-ounce) cartons low-fat lemon yogurt
1/4 cup blanched almonds, chopped and toasted
1 teaspoon grated orange rind
2 tablespoons orange juice

Combine the lemon yogurt, almonds, orange rind, and orange juice and mix well. Refrigerate. Keeps in refrigerator 1 week.

Nutritional information per serving

Calories 88, Protein (g) 4, Carbohydrate (g) 10, Fat (g) 3, Cal. from Fat (%) 30, Saturated Fat (g) 1, Dietary Fiber (g) 1, Cholesterol (mg) 3, Sodium (mg) 38, Diabetic Exchanges: 0.5 skim milk, 0.5 fat

DOC'S NOTES:

Yogurt is an excellent source of calcium and protein, and a good source of riboflavin, phosphorus and Vitamin B12.

Strawberry Salsa 🥕

A great dip or complement to whatever you serve such as chicken or fish.

MAKES EIGHT (1/4-CUP) SERVINGS

2 cups strawberries
1/2 cup chopped green bell peppers
2 tablespoons chopped red onion
2 tablespoons chopped parsley
2 tablespoons raspberry vinegar
1 tablespoon canola oil
1 tablespoon honey
Dash of hot pepper sauce, optional
Tortilla chips

In a bowl, combine strawberries, green pepper, onions, and parsley. In a separate bowl, combine vinegar, oil, honey, and hot sauce. Toss with strawberry mixture. Cover and refrigerate for 2 hours. Serve with tortilla chips.

Nutritional information per serving

Calories 38, Protein (g) 0, Carbohydrate (g) 6, Fat (g) 2, Cal. from Fat (%) 41, Saturated Fat (g) 0, Dietary Fiber (g) 1, Cholesterol (mg) 0, Sodium (mg) 1, Diabetic Exchanges: 0.5 fruit, 0.5 fat

DOC'S NOTES:

Not only is this delicious it is also a good source of Vitamin C and potassium.

Artichoke Squares 🥕

Great served warm, room temperature, or cold, and very appealing.

MAKES 35 SQUARES

1 cup chopped green onions (scallions)
1 teaspoon minced garlic
2 cups sliced mushrooms
1 (2 ounce) jar diced pimentos, drained
2 (14-ounce) cans artichoke hearts,
   drained and chopped
1/4 cup chopped parsley
1/2 teaspoon dried oregano leaves
2 large eggs
3 large egg whites
3/4 cup Italian bread crumbs
1 cup shredded reduced-fat Swiss cheese
1 cup shredded reduced-fat Cheddar cheese
Salt and pepper to taste

Preheat oven to 350 degrees. In pan coated with nonstick cooking spray, sauté onion, garlic, and mushrooms until tender. In a bowl, combine onion mixture, pimentos, artichoke hearts, parsley, oregano, egg, egg whites, bread crumbs, cheeses, salt and pepper, mixing well. Pour into a 13×9×2-inch baking dish coated with nonstick cooking spray and bake for 30 minutes or until mixture is set. Cut into squares.

Nutritional information per serving
Calories 43, Protein (g) 3, Carbohydrate (g) 3,
Fat (g) 2, Cal. from Fat (%) 37, Saturated Fat (g) 1,
Dietary Fiber (g) 1, Cholesterol (mg) 16, Sodium (mg) 137,
Diabetic Exchanges: 0.5 lean meat

DOC'S NOTES:

Artichokes provide Vitamin C, folacin, magnesium, phosphorus, and potassium. Mushrooms provide B Vitamins, copper, and other minerals.

Italian Pasta Salad 🥕

This vegetarian salad can be adjusted to your taste and your pantry. Use your imagination and your favorite kind of pasta.

MAKES **8** TO **12** SERVINGS

8 ounces ziti pasta

4 ounces tri-colored rotini

1 green bell pepper, cored and chopped

1 red bell pepper, cored and chopped

1/2 cup chopped celery

2 teaspoons drained capers

1/3 cup chopped green onions (scallions)

2 Roma (plum) tomatoes, chopped

1/2 cup red wine vinegar

1/4 cup water

1 teaspoon dried basil leaves

1 teaspoon dried oregano leaves

1/2 teaspoon minced garlic

1 tablespoon Dijon mustard

1/4 cup grated Parmesan cheese

Cook both the pastas together according to package directions, omitting the oil and salt. Rinse and drain and place in a large bowl. Add the bell peppers, celery, capers, green onions, and tomatoes. Combine the vinegar with the water, basil, oregano, garlic, mustard, and Parmesan cheese in a small bowl, mixing well. Pour over the pasta mixture and toss well. Serve or refrigerate.

Nutritional information per serving
Calories 127, Protein (g) 5, Carbohydrate (g) 24, Fat (g) 1, Cal. from Fat (%) 8, Saturated Fat (g) 1, Dietary Fiber (g) 1, Cholesterol (mg) 2, Sodium (mg) 96, Diabetic Exchanges: 1.5 starch

DOC'S NOTES:

Pasta is rich in complex carbohydrates, high in protein, low in fat and delicious.

Mini Cheese Pizzas ✏️ ❄️

These are easy to make and are super for a quick snack or lunch.

MAKES 10 PIZZAS

1 (10-biscuit) can flaky refrigerated biscuits
⅓ cup tomato sauce
½ teaspoon dried oregano leaves
½ cup shredded part-skim Mozzarella cheese

Preheat oven to 450 degrees. Pat each biscuit into a 4-inch circle on a baking sheet coated with nonstick cooking spray. In a small bowl, mix together the tomato sauce and oregano. Spoon the sauce on each biscuit round. Sprinkle the cheese over the tomato sauce. Bake for 8 to 10 minutes or until the cheese is melted.

Nutritional information per serving
Calories 117, Protein (g) 4, Carbohydrate (g) 15,
Fat (g) 5, Cal. from Fat (%) 40, Saturated Fat (g) 2,
Dietary Fiber (g) 0, Cholesterol (mg) 3, Sodium (mg) 424,
Diabetic Exchanges: 1 starch, 1 fat

DOC'S NOTES:

Add appealing veggies for extra nutrition.

Fresh Tomato and Cheese Pizza 🥕

Simply tomato and cheese, yet interesting enough to enjoy.

MAKES 8 SLICES

2 thin slices red onion, cut in half
2 cloves garlic, thinly sliced
1 (10-ounce) can refrigerated pizza crust dough
  or Boboli prepared crust
1 (15-ounce) carton nonfat ricotta cheese
1 cup shredded part-skim mozzarella cheese
1/4 cup grated Parmesan cheese, divided
1 tablespoon dried basil leaves
4 Roma (plum) tomatoes, thinly sliced

Preheat the broiler. Place the onion and garlic on a baking sheet coated with nonstick cooking spray. Broil 6 inches from the heat 8 to 10 minutes, or until charred; set aside. Change oven setting to bake at 450 degrees.

Roll the dough into a 12-inch circle and press into a pizza pan coated with nonstick cooking spray.

Combine the ricotta cheese, mozzarella cheese, Parmesan cheese, and basil, stirring well. Spread the cheese over the dough, leaving a 1/2-inch border. Arrange the tomato slices over the cheese. Top with the onion and garlic.

Bake on the bottom rack of the oven for 10 to 12 minutes, or until the crust is browned. Transfer the pizza to a cutting board.

Nutritional information per serving

Calories 184, Protein (g) 15, Carbohydrate (g) 20, Fat (g) 5, Cal. from Fat (%) 22, Saturated Fat (g) 2, Dietary Fiber (g) 1, Cholesterol (mg) 15, Sodium (mg) 445, Diabetic Exchanges: 1.5 lean meat, 1 starch, 1 vegetable

DOC'S NOTES:

Italian food seems to be a favorite among patients receiving chemotherapy. As long as your mouth is not sore and your white blood cell count is not low, enjoy! The cheese provides protein and calcium while the tomatoes are rich in vitamins A and C.

Asparagus and Brie Pizza ✏ ❄

By using asparagus and Brie you turn this ordinary pizza into something special.

MAKES 8 SLICES

12 thin asparagus spears, tips only
1 red bell pepper, cored and thinly sliced, optional
1 teaspoon minced garlic
1 (10-ounce) can refrigerated pizza crust or
    1 (16-ounce) Boboli prepared crust
1/2 teaspoon dried basil leaves
1/2 teaspoon dried oregano leaves
Salt and pepper to taste
3 1/2 ounces Brie cheese, skin removed and
    thinly sliced

Preheat oven to 425 degrees. Cook the asparagus tips in a small pot with 1/2 cup water or cook in microwave until tender. Drain and set aside. Heat a skillet coated with nonstick cooking spray over medium heat and sauté the bell pepper until tender, about 4 minutes. Blend in the garlic.

Coat a 12-inch pizza pan with nonstick cooking spray. Unroll the dough and place in the prepared pan, starting at the center and pressing out with your hands. Bake for 5 minutes. Remove and sprinkle the crust with the basil, oregano, and salt and pepper. Then evenly distribute the Brie cheese, bell pepper, and asparagus on top. Bake for 8 to 10 minutes more.

Nutritional information per serving
Calories 133, Protein (g) 6, Carbohydrate (g) 17, Fat (g) 5, Cal. from Fat (%) 31, Saturated Fat (g) 2, Dietary Fiber (g) 1, Cholesterol (mg) 12, Sodium (mg) 294, Diabetic Exchanges: 0.5 lean meat, 1 starch, 0.5 fat

DOC'S NOTES:

Asparagus is rich in Vitamins A, B6, C, and E. It also has a high content of folacin.

SNACKS AND LIGHT MEALS

Spinach and Cheese Tortilla Pizza 🥕

By using tortillas, this is an easy yet satisfying meal.

MAKES 12 SLICES

2 large (10-inch) flour tortillas
2 tablespoons nonfat plain yogurt
1 (10-ounce) package frozen chopped spinach, thawed and squeezed dry
1 large tomato, chopped
½ cup shredded reduced-fat Monterey Jack cheese
¼ cup chopped green onions (scallions)

Preheat oven to 450 degrees. Place the tortillas on a baking sheet coated with nonstick cooking spray. Bake for 3 minutes, or until golden brown. Remove from the oven and reduce the temperature to 350 degrees. Spread the yogurt evenly over the tortillas. Top with the spinach and tomato. Next, sprinkle evenly with the Monterey Jack cheese. Bake for 5 minutes more, or until the cheese is melted. Sprinkle with the green onions. Cut each tortilla into 6 slices and serve immediately.

Nutritional information per serving

Calories 64, Protein (g) 3, Carbohydrate (g) 9, Fat (g) 2, Cal. from Fat (%) 25, Saturated Fat (g) 1, Dietary Fiber (g) 1, Cholesterol (mg) 3, Sodium (mg) 108, Diabetic Exchanges: 0.5 starch

DOC'S NOTES:

You will have to fight your family for these. Spinach is a great source of beta carotene and folate.

Cheese Quesadillas ✎ ❄

Add sautéed veggies or keep it simple with cheese for this simple snack or meal.

MAKES 6 SLICES

2 (8-inch) flour tortillas
1/2 cup shredded reduced-fat Cheddar or Monterey
  Jack cheese
Taco sauce

In a pan coated with nonstick cooking spray, on a low heat, place one flour tortilla. Sprinkle with the cheese and top with the other flour tortilla. Cook about 1 to 1 1/2 minutes on each side turning with a spatula. Coat the pan again with nonstick cooking spray before turning over. Make sure the cheese is melted and the tortillas are light brown. Watch carefully and cook slowly over a low heat to allow the cheese to melt. Cut into wedges and serve with taco sauce.

Nutritional information per serving
Calories 80, Protein (g) 4, Carbohydrate (g) 9,
Fat (g) 3, Cal. from Fat (%) 33, Saturated Fat (g) 2,
Dietary Fiber (g) 1, Cholesterol (mg) 5, Sodium (mg) 138,
Diabetic Exchanges: 0.5 lean meat, 0.5 starch

DOC'S NOTES:

Add leftover veggies to increase the nutritional value.

Italian Spinach Pie 🥕

A quiche-like pie that makes a light meal.

MAKES 6 SERVINGS

½ cup chopped onions
2 (10-ounce) packages frozen chopped spinach
1 (14½-ounce) can artichoke hearts, quartered
1 cup fat-free ricotta cheese
¼ cup skim milk
2 large egg whites, beaten with a fork
½ teaspoon garlic powder
1 (8-ounce) can no-salt added tomato sauce
½ teaspoon dried oregano leaves
½ teaspoon dried basil leaves
½ cup shredded part-skim mozzarella cheese

Preheat oven to 350 degrees. In a skillet coated with nonstick cooking spray, sauté the onions over medium heat until tender, about 5 minutes. Meanwhile, cook the spinach according to package directions; drain very well. In a large bowl, combine the onions, spinach, artichoke hearts, ricotta cheese, milk, egg whites, and garlic powder, mixing well. Spoon the mixture into a 9-inch pie plate coated with nonstick cooking spray. Mix the tomato sauce with the oregano and basil and spread evenly over the spinach. Bake for 15 minutes. Sprinkle with the mozzarella cheese and bake for 5 to 10 minutes longer, until the cheese is melted.

Nutritional information per serving
Calories 116, Protein (g) 14, Carbohydrate (g) 12,
Fat (g) 2, Cal. from Fat (%) 14, Saturated Fat (g) 1,
Dietary Fiber (g) 4, Cholesterol (mg) 9, Sodium (mg) 342,
Diabetic Exchanges: 1.5 very lean meat, 2 vegetable0

DOC'S NOTES:

Spinach provides potassium while the tomatoes add vitamins A and C, folacin, magnesium, phosphorus, and potassium.

Southwestern Stuffed Potatoes 🥕 ❄️

This variation is a great choice if you enjoy stuffed potatoes. Make a bunch and freeze for a quick lunch.

MAKES 6 SERVINGS

3 medium baking potatoes
3 tablespoons margarine
2 tablespoons skim milk
1/2 cup nonfat plain yogurt
1 1/2 cups frozen corn, thawed
1 (4-ounce) can diced green chiles, optional
4 green onions (scallions), chopped
1 cup shredded reduced-fat Cheddar cheese
Paprika

Preheat oven to 400 degrees. Wash potatoes well, and dry thoroughly. With fork, prick skins over entire surface. Place potatoes directly on oven rack, and bake for about 1 hour or until soft when squeezed. When done, cut each potato in half lengthwise. Scoop out inside, leaving a thin shell. In mixer, mash potato pulp until no lumps remain. Add margarine, skim milk, and yogurt, mixing well. Stir in corn, green chiles, green onions, and cheese, combining well. Spoon mixture into shells. Top with paprika. Lower oven to 350 degrees and bake for about 20 minutes or until cheese is melted and potatoes are hot.

Nutritional information per serving
Calories 222, Protein (g) 10, Carbohydrate (g) 26, Fat (g) 9, Cal. from Fat (%) 37, Saturated Fat (g) 3, Dietary Fiber (g) 3, Cholesterol (mg) 11, Sodium (mg) 213, Diabetic Exchanges: 1 lean meat, 2 starch, 1 fat

DOC'S NOTES:

Potatoes stuffed with corn and cheese offer health benefits besides a great snack to pop in the microwave.

Coffee Cake 🥕 ❄️

This cake will definitely be a hit for all those coffee cake lovers.

MAKES 24 SERVINGS

1 (8-ounce) tub margarine
1¼ cups sugar
2 cups nonfat plain yogurt
3 large egg whites
1 teaspoon vanilla extract
1 teaspoon imitation butter flavoring
3 cups all-purpose flour
1½ teaspoons baking powder
1 teaspoon baking soda

Preheat oven to 350 degrees. In mixing bowl, beat margarine and sugar until fluffy. Add yogurt, egg whites, vanilla, and butter flavoring, mixing well. Combine flour, baking powder, and baking soda together. Gradually add to yogurt mixture, mixing well. Pour one third of the batter into a 10-inch Bundt pan coated with nonstick cooking spray and dusted with flour. Sprinkle with half the Nut Filling (recipe follows). Repeat layers, ending with batter. Bake for 55 minutes or until toothpick inserted in center of cake comes out clean.

NUT FILLING

½ cup light brown sugar
1½ teaspoons ground cinnamon
½ cup chopped pecans

In a small bowl, combine all ingredients. Mix with fork until crumbly.

Nutritional information per serving
Calories 214, Protein (g) 4, Carbohydrate (g) 29, Fat (g) 9, Cal. from Fat (%) 39, Saturated Fat (g) 2, Dietary Fiber (g) 1, Cholesterol (mg) 0, Sodium (mg) 179, Diabetic Exchanges: 1 starch, 1 other carb., 1.5 fat

DOC'S NOTES:

An easy morning or afternoon pick up snack.

SNACKS AND
LIGHT MEALS

No Bake Cookies 🥕

These ingredients are always in the pantry. A quick and nourishing cure for a sweet tooth.

MAKES 3 TO 3½ DOZEN

½ cup graham cracker crumbs
2½ cups old fashioned oatmeal
½ cup sugar
2 tablespoons cocoa
½ cup skim milk
½ cup margarine
½ cup reduced-fat peanut butter
1 teaspoon vanilla extract

In a bowl, combine graham cracker crumbs and oatmeal. Set aside. In a saucepan, stir sugar, cocoa, milk, and margarine over medium heat until dissolved. Bring mixture to a boil and cook for 2 minutes. Remove from heat. Stir in peanut butter and vanilla until well combined. Quickly blend in cracker mixture. Beat by hand for a few minutes or until thickened. Drop by teaspoonfuls onto waxed paper. Refrigerate until firm and store in refrigerator.

Nutritional information per serving
Calories 71, Protein (g) 2, Carbohydrate (g) 8,
Fat (g) 4, Cal. from Fat (%) 46, Saturated Fat (g) 1,
Dietary Fiber (g) 1, Cholesterol (mg) 0, Sodium (mg) 57,
Diabetic Exchanges: 0.5 starch, 1 fat

DOC'S NOTES:

These cookies are a good source of fiber and protein. Peanuts are a good source of thiamin, niacin, folacin, iron, and magnesium.

Mocha Meringue Mounds 🥕

Meringues with lots of personality! These are easy to tolerate.

Makes 3 dozen meringue mounds

3 large egg whites
Dash of salt
½ cup sugar
1 tablespoon instant coffee
½ teaspoon vanilla extract
½ cup mini semisweet chocolate chips

Preheat oven to 300 degrees. In a large mixing bowl, beat egg whites with dash of salt at high speed of mixer for one minute. Mix sugar with instant coffee, and gradually add sugar mixture, 1 tablespoon at a time, beating 3 minutes or until stiff peaks form and sugar mixture is dissolved. Beat in vanilla. Gently fold in chocolate chips. Drop by heaping teaspoonfuls onto a baking sheet lined with wax paper. Bake for 30 minutes. Cool slightly on baking sheet before removing.

Nutritional information per serving

Calories 24, Protein (g) 0, Carbohydrate (g) 4, Fat (g) 1, Cal. from Fat (%) 25, Saturated Fat (g) 0, Dietary Fiber (g) 0, Cholesterol (mg) 0, Sodium (mg) 5, Diabetic Exchanges: 0.5 other carb.

DOC'S NOTES:

No fat or cholesterol, these are perfect pop-in-the-mouth, light snacks.

- ✦ Should frozen dishes be brought over?
- ✦ Are snacks a good idea?

There is nothing more comforting when you are sick than an act of kindness from a friend. Sometimes patients do not want to discuss their appetite or their situation. Being there to listen and offer a warm smile is often the greatest gift. A thoughtful snack, casserole, or other healthy dish can bring joy and happiness to a loved one. This can also be helpful for family members or caregivers.

Even the smell of cooking can upset your stomach at times. Patients tell me that often they have their food prepared in an outside kitchen to avoid the aroma. Having a surprise will sometimes entice you to eat. We will try to offer recipes for foods and drinks that can be heated, defrosted, or served with minimal preparation. A real treat is to include paper plates, forks and spoons so you do not have to worry about washing dishes and your meal really is ready to eat. Try to keep it simple and inviting. Eating with a friend or family can also be very helpful. It is no fun to eat alone.

What Can People Do To Help?
- ✦ Encourage and support without being overwhelming.
- ✦ Accompany you to the grocery store.
- ✦ Take your list and go shopping for you.
- ✦ Help you to prepare food.
- ✦ Help organize ready-to-eat snacks.
- ✦ Organize friends/or relatives to cook for you and your family.
- ✦ Meals should be brought over in disposable containers.
- ✦ Run errands for you.
- ✦ Eat with you.
- ✦ Take you for a ride.
- ✦ Read to you.
- ✦ Give the caregiver a break.

Banana Bread

I hate the thought of throwing bananas away so when I have ripe bananas I always make a banana bread and stick it in my freezer to pull out or bring to a friend. For added calories and taste, add some chocolate chips or butterscotch chips.

MAKES 16 SLICES

1/3 cup canola oil
1 cup dark brown sugar
2 large eggs
3 medium bananas, mashed
1 teaspoon vanilla extract
2 cups all-purpose flour
1 teaspoon baking soda
1 teaspoon ground cinnamon

Preheat oven to 350 degrees. In a mixing bowl, beat together the oil and brown sugar. Add eggs, banana, and vanilla. In a separate bowl, combine flour, baking soda and cinnamon. Gradually add the dry ingredients, stirring until mixed. Pour batter into a 9×5×3-inch loaf pan coated with nonstick cooking spray. Bake 50 to 60 minutes or until a toothpick inserted in the center comes out clean.

Nutritional information per serving
Calories 180, Protein (g) 3, Carbohydrate (g) 31, Fat (g) 5, Cal. from Fat (%) 27, Saturated Fat (g) 1, Dietary Fiber (g) 1, Cholesterol (mg) 27, Sodium (mg) 93, Diabetic Exchanges: 1 starch, 0.5 fruit, 0.5 other carb., 1 fat

DOC'S NOTES:

Banana Bread is great for an afternoon snack or a light breakfast. The bananas are a good food to consume if diarrhea is a problem. Each banana has about 450 mg of potassium.

Spinach
Layered Dish 🥕

Prepare the night before to enjoy the next day for brunch or a light dinner. Spinach and a light red sauce layered with cheese.

MAKES 10 TO 12 SERVINGS

1/2 pound mushrooms, sliced

1 onion, chopped

1 teaspoon minced garlic, divided

1 (10-ounce) package frozen chopped spinach, thawed and squeezed dry

1 (28-ounce) can crushed tomatoes with their juice

1 teaspoon dried oregano leaves

12 slices Italian bread, crusts removed

1 (8-ounce) package part-skim Mozzarella cheese, shredded

4 large eggs

4 large egg whites

2 cups skim milk

In a medium skillet coated with nonstick cooking spray, sauté the mushrooms, onion, and 1/2 teaspoon garlic until tender, about 3 to 5 minutes. Add the spinach, mixing well; set aside. In a small bowl, mix together the tomatoes, oregano, and remaining 1/2 teaspoon garlic. Spread about 1 cup of the tomato sauce along the bottom of a 3-quart casserole dish coated with nonstick cooking spray. Top with 6 slices of the bread. Cover the bread evenly with half of the spinach mixture, half the cheese, and another 1 cup of the sauce. Repeat the layers with the remaining bread, spinach, cheese, and sauce. In a separate bowl or in a food processor, whisk or blend together the eggs, egg whites and skim milk. Pour the egg mixture slowly over the casserole until the mixture has been absorbed. Cover and refrigerate for 6 hours or overnight. Preheat oven to 350 degrees. Place the casserole in the oven and bake for 1 hour or until all the egg mixture is done.

Nutritional information per serving

Calories 184, Protein (g) 14, Carbohydrate (g) 21, Fat (g) 6, Cal. from Fat (%) 28, Saturated Fat (g) 3, Dietary Fiber (g) 3, Cholesterol (mg) 83, Sodium (mg) 371, Diabetic Exchanges: 1 lean meat, 0.5 starch, 2 vegetable, 0.5 fat

DOC'S NOTES:

The tomatoes may be a little rough on a sore mouth, but if your mouth feels good, enjoy. Eggs provide a good source of high quality protein and are an important source of Vitamins B12 and E, riboflavin, folacin, iron, and phosphorus. Spinach is high in beta carotene, iron, and calcium.

CAREGIVER

Breakfast Casserole 🥕

This egg dish is always a hit and can be prepared ahead of time. Bringing over uncooked is also an option. Remember, if you prepare the casserole in a glass dish, place in a cold oven, then turn the oven on and add 10 to 15 minutes longer to the baking time.

MAKES **12** SERVINGS

8 slices of white bread, crust removed

3 ounces Canadian bacon, chopped

1 bunch green onions (scallions), chopped

2 cups broccoli florets

5 large eggs, beaten

3 large egg whites

2½ cups skim milk

1 teaspoon dry mustard

1 cup nonfat plain yogurt

½ cup grated Parmesan cheese

½ teaspoon minced garlic

2 tablespoons chopped parsley

1 teaspoon dried basil leaves

1 tablespoon dried rosemary leaves

Salt and pepper to taste

Arrange the bread along the bottom of a 3-quart oblong casserole dish or a 13×9×2-inch baking pan, overlapping the slices slightly. In a small skillet coated with nonstick cooking spray, sauté the bacon, green onions, and broccoli over medium heat until tender, about 8 minutes. Spread on top of the bread. In a mixing bowl, blend the eggs, egg whites, skim milk, and mustard; set aside. In a food processor, blend the yogurt, Parmesan cheese, garlic, parsley, basil, rosemary, and salt and pepper. Pour into the egg mixture, stirring until well combined. Pour over the bread and press the bread down to soak up the liquid. Cover with plastic wrap and place in the refrigerator for at least 6 hours or overnight. Preheat oven to 375 degrees. Bake for 1 hour, or until browned and a knife inserted in the center comes out clean.

Nutritional information per serving

Calories 150, Protein (g) 12, Carbohydrate (g) 15, Fat (g) 5, Cal. from Fat (%) 29, Saturated Fat (g) 2, Dietary Fiber (g) 1, Cholesterol (mg) 97, Sodium (mg) 358, Diabetic Exchanges: 1 lean meat, 0.5 starch, 0.5 skim milk

DOC'S NOTES:

Bring to a friend the night before so it can be enjoyed freshly baked the next morning or for a light dinner. Whole wheat bread can be substituted for the white bread. This dish is high in protein and contains a cruciferous vegetable.

CAREGIVER

Cauliflower Soup 🥕 ❄️

Throw all the ingredients into a food processor to blend a smooth, creamy soup; great serve hot or cold.

MAKES SIX (1-CUP) SERVINGS

4 cups cooked cauliflower flowerets
1/2 cup shredded reduced fat Cheddar cheese
1 tablespoon all-purpose flour
1 1/3 cups buttermilk
1 cup canned fat-free chicken broth
1 clove garlic, minced
Salt and pepper to taste

Place all ingredients in a food processor or blender and process until smooth. Serve immediately or refrigerate if serving cold, heat if soup is to be served hot. Add more broth as needed to thin.

Nutritional information per serving
Calories 76, Protein (g) 7, Carbohydrate (g) 7, Fat (g) 3, Cal. from Fat (%) 29, Saturated Fat (g) 2, Dietary Fiber (g) 2, Cholesterol (mg) 7, Sodium (mg) 233, Diabetic Exchanges: 0.5 lean meat, 1 vegetable

DOC'S NOTES:

Cauliflower is a cruciferous vegetable which can help reduce the risk of cancer.

Quick Cheesy Potato Soup 🥕 ❄️

If you don't like to cook, this easy recipe for a favorite velvety soup is for you.

MAKES SIX (1-CUP) SERVINGS

1 large onion
2 carrots, peeled
1 green bell pepper, cored
2 (10 3/4-ounce) cans cream of potato soup
2 cups chicken broth
2 ounces pasteurized processed light
   cheese spread
1 (8-ounce) carton nonfat plain yogurt

Chop the onion, carrots, and green bell pepper in a food processor. In a large pot coated with nonstick cooking spray, sauté the chopped vegetables over medium heat until tender, about 5 minutes. Add the soup, chicken broth, and cheese, stirring until the cheese is melted and the soup is well heated. Before serving, stir in the yogurt; do not boil.

Nutritional information per serving
Calories 131, Protein (g) 7, Carbohydrate (g) 20, Fat (g) 3, Cal. from Fat (%) 21, Saturated Fat (g) 1, Dietary Fiber (g) 2, Cholesterol (mg) 9, Sodium (mg) 1132, Diabetic Exchanges: 0.5 starch, 2 vegetable, 0.5 fat

CAREGIVER

Quick and Easy Corn and Shrimp Soup ✳

This delicious, easy recipe is a winner. Take to a friend in plastic containers with the green onions in a separate bag. They can serve immediately or freeze. I always double this recipe as it is a family favorite.

Makes 8 servings

1 onion, chopped

1 teaspoon minced garlic

1 green bell pepper, cored and chopped

1 (8-ounce) package fat-free cream cheese, softened

2 (10¾-ounce) cans cream of shrimp soup or corn chowder soup or combination

2 (14¾-ounce) cans cream- style corn

2 cups skim milk

1 (10-ounce) can diced tomatoes and green chiles

1 pound medium shrimp, peeled

Chopped green onions, optional

In a heavy large pot, coated with nonstick cooking spray, sauté onion, garlic, and green pepper until tender, about 5 minutes. Stir in cream cheese. Add soup, cream-style corn, milk, tomatoes, and shrimp. Bring to a boil, reduce heat, and cook until shrimp are done, about 7 to 10 minutes. Serve with green onions. When reheating soup, if too thick, add more milk.

Nutritional information per serving

Calories 283, Protein (g) 20, Carbohydrate (g) 41, Fat (g) 4, Cal. from Fat (%) 16, Saturated Fat (g) 2, Dietary Fiber (g) 2, Cholesterol (mg) 94, Sodium (mg) 1528, Diabetic Exchanges: 1 lean meat, 2 starch, 1 vegetable, 0.5 skim milk

DOC'S NOTES:

A cup of this soup will be a great addition to any meal or a complete meal in itself. Low in fat, high in fiber and Vitamin A. Vitamin A helps generate pigment necessary for the proper workings of the retina. It also helps form and maintain healthy skin, teeth, mucous membranes, and skeletal and soft tissue.

Cream of Spinach Soup 🥕 ❄️

Frozen broccoli can also be used for a broccoli soup version. For soup craving, here's an easy idea. Soups are enjoyed any time of day and freeze well.

MAKES EIGHT (1-CUP) SERVINGS

1/2 pound fresh mushrooms, sliced
1 small onion, chopped
2 (10³/4-ounce) cans reduced-fat cream of mushroom soup
1³/4 cups canned fat-free chicken broth or vegetable broth
2 (10-ounce) packages frozen chopped spinach, cooked according to package directions and drained well
Salt and pepper to taste

In a large pot coated with nonstick cooking spray, sauté the mushrooms and onion until tender over medium heat for 5 minutes. Add the soup, chicken broth, spinach, and salt and pepper, stirring until thoroughly heated. Transfer to a food processor or blender to purée.

Nutritional information per serving
Calories 76, Protein (g) 4, Carbohydrate (g) 11, Fat (g) 2, Cal. from Fat (%) 24, Saturated Fat (g) 1, Dietary Fiber (g) 3, Cholesterol (mg) 3, Sodium (mg) 700, Diabetic Exchanges: 0.5 starch, 1 vegetable, 0.5 fat

DOC'S NOTES:

Mushrooms are a good source of B vitamins, copper and other vitamins. Spinach is a good source of vitamins and rich source of beta carotene, protein, and folacin. Folacin is important in the synthesis of DNA, which controls cell function. Folacin acts with B12 to produce red blood cells.

CAREGIVER

Chicken Tortilla Soup ❄

Popular and a really tasty version of chicken soup. Bring the condiments over in zip-top bags. Use different flavored tortillas to make the tortilla strips and make extras to have for snacks.

MAKES 6 TO 8 SERVINGS

SOUP

1 onion, chopped
1 teaspoon minced garlic
4 cups canned fat-free chicken broth
1 (28-ounce) can diced tomatoes
1½ pounds boneless skinless chicken breasts, cut into chunks
1 tablespoon chili powder
1 teaspoon ground cumin
2 tablespoon lime juice
1 (16-ounce) bag frozen corn

TORTILLA STRIPS AND CONDIMENTS

6 (8-inch) flour tortillas, baked
1 cup shredded reduced-fat Cheddar cheese
½ cup chopped green onions (scallions)
1 small avocado, peeled and diced, optional

In a large pot coated with nonstick cooking spray, sauté the onion and garlic until tender, about 5 minutes. Add the chicken broth, tomatoes, chicken, chili powder, cumin, and lime juice; bring mixture to a boil. Lower heat and continue cooking until chicken is done, about 17 to 20 minutes. Add corn and continue cooking 5 more minutes. Serve with tortilla strips and condiments.

To make tortilla strips, while soup is cooking, preheat oven to 350 degrees. Cut tortillas into ½-inch wide strips. Coat a baking sheet with nonstick cooking spray and lay strips over sheet. Bake 15 to 20 minutes or until lightly browned. Strips may be stored in zip-top bags.

Nutritional information per serving
Calories 345, Protein (g) 31, Carbohydrate (g) 40, Fat (g) 7, Cal. from Fat (%) 18, Saturated Fat (g) 3, Dietary Fiber (g) 5, Cholesterol (mg) 57, Sodium (mg) 791, Diabetic Exchanges: 2.5 lean meat, 2 starch, 2 vegetable

DOC'S NOTES:

A dish your whole family will enjoy. Tomatoes are high in lypocene, and Vitamins A and C. Vitamin C is a member of the antioxidant family of vitamins. Vitamin C promotes healthy gums and teeth, aiding in iron absorption and wound healing.

Rice Taco Salad

I like to add additional beans, corn and avocado for more nutritional benefits and because these are some of my favorite ingredients. This salad is appealing to all ages and is hearty enough for a satisfying meal.

MAKES 6 SERVINGS

1 pound ground sirloin
1/2 cup finely chopped onion
1 clove garlic, minced
1/2 teaspoon ground cumin
Salt and pepper to taste
3 cups cooked rice
4 cups mixed greens
2 tomatoes, chopped
1/2 cup shredded reduced-fat Cheddar cheese
1/3 cup nonfat plain yogurt
1/3 cup picante sauce
Low-fat tortilla chips, optional

In a large skillet coated with nonstick cooking spray, cook the beef, onion, and garlic over medium heat, stirring to crumble, about 5 to 7 minutes, or until the meat is done. Drain any excess fat. Add the cumin, salt and pepper, and rice. Remove from the heat and let cool. In a large bowl, combine the greens, tomatoes, cheese, and rice mixture. In a small bowl, mix together the yogurt and picante sauce and toss with salad when serving. Serve immediately with tortilla chips, if desired.

Nutritional information per serving

Calories 250, Protein (g) 21, Carbohydrate (g) 29, Fat (g) 5, Cal. from Fat (%) 20, Saturated Fat (g) 3, Dietary Fiber (g) 2, Cholesterol (mg) 45, Sodium (mg) 243, Diabetic Exchanges: 2.5 lean meat, 1.5 starch, 1.5 vegetable

DOC'S NOTES:

Try using brown rice for extra fiber.

CAREGIVER

Manicotti ❄

This one dish meal featuring spinach, meat, and cheese freezes well also.

MAKES 8 SERVINGS

1 (8-ounce) package manicotti shells
1 pound ground sirloin
1/2 cup chopped onion
1 teaspoon minced garlic
1 cup reduced-fat ricotta cheese
1 (8-ounce) package reduced-fat cream cheese
1 (10-ounce) package frozen chopped spinach,
   thawed and squeezed dry
1 (28-ounce) can chopped tomatoes,
   in own juices
1 teaspoon dried oregano leaves
1 teaspoon dried basil leaves
Salt and pepper to taste

Preheat oven to 350 degrees. Cook the manicotti shells according to package directions, omitting any oil and salt. Rinse, drain, and set aside. In a large skillet coated with nonstick cooking spray, cook the meat, onion, and garlic until the meat is done, about 7 minutes; drain any excess grease. Mix in the ricotta, cream cheese, and spinach. Stuff the shells with the meat mixture and arrange in a baking dish coated with nonstick cooking spray.

In a separate bowl, combine the tomatoes, oregano, basil, salt and pepper. Pour over the shells. Cover and bake for 15 minutes. Uncover and bake for 10 minutes longer, or until bubbly and well heated.

Nutrition information per serving
Calories 330, Protein (g) 23m, Carbohydrate (g) 36, Fat (g) 11, Calories from Fat (%) 29, Saturated Fat (g) 6, Dietary Fiber (g) 4, Cholesterol (mg) 58, Sodium (mg) 337, Diabetic Exchanges: 2.5 lean meat, 2 starch, 1.5 vegetable

DOC'S NOTES:

This antioxidant rich recipe includes spinach, high in folate, and tomatoes, high in lycopene, all which can reduce cancer.

Company Chicken ❄

This fabulous tasting dish and sauce puts it high on any list. Bring a zip-top bag of wild rice, also. This dish also freezes well.

MAKES 6 SERVINGS

2 pounds boneless skinless chicken breasts
Salt and pepper to taste
2 tablespoons margarine
½ pound mushrooms, sliced
½ cup sherry or chicken broth
2 tablespoons lemon juice
1 (14-ounce) can artichokes, drained
1 cup evaporated skimmed milk
½ cup chopped green onion (scallions) stems
½ cup nonfat plain yogurt

Season the chicken breasts with salt and pepper. In a large skillet coated with nonstick cooking spray, heat the margarine until melted. Brown the chicken on both sides, about 3 to 5 minutes on each side. Add the mushrooms, sherry, and lemon juice. Bring to a boil, reduce the heat and cover, for 20 to 30 minutes or until chicken is done. Add the artichokes and milk, stirring and cooking for 5 more minutes. Stir in the green onion stems and yogurt. Do not boil.

Nutritional information per serving
Calories 287, Protein (g) 42, Carbohydrate (g) 12, Fat (g) 6, Cal. from Fat (%) 19, Saturated Fat (g) 1, Dietary Fiber (g) 1, Cholesterol (mg) 90, Sodium (mg) 330, Diabetic Exchanges: 4 lean meat, 0.5 skim milk, 1 vegetable

DOC'S NOTES:

Company Chicken with a salad is a complete meal. High in B Vitamins, copper, and other minerals. B vitamins help convert carbohydrates into energy. A deficiency of B vitamins can cause skin to become dry and cracked.

CAREGIVER

Mexican Chicken Casserole ❄

A layered Mexican casserole that will be appreciated by all. For a less spicy version, use plain tomatoes.

MAKES 8 SERVINGS

1½ cups canned fat-free chicken broth
1 cup skim milk
½ cup all-purpose flour
½ cup nonfat plain yogurt
1 (10-ounce) can diced tomatoes and green
    chiles, drained
¼ cup chopped parsley
1 tablespoon chili powder
1 teaspoon dried oregano leaves
Salt and pepper to taste
1 onion, chopped
1 green bell pepper, cored and chopped
2 cloves garlic, minced
10 flour tortillas, cut in quarters
2 cups skinless cooked chicken breast chunks
½ cup shredded reduced-fat sharp
    Cheddar cheese

Preheat oven to 350 degrees. In saucepan, bring chicken broth to a simmer. In small bowl, whisk milk into flour to make a smooth paste. Add to chicken broth and cook until thickened and smooth, stirring constantly. Remove from heat and stir in yogurt, tomatoes, parsley, chili powder, and oregano.

Season with salt and pepper to taste; set aside. In skillet coated with nonstick cooking spray, sauté onions, green pepper, and garlic until tender. Line bottom of a shallow 3-quart baking dish with half the tortillas. Sprinkle half of the chicken and half of the onion mixture over the tortillas. Spoon half of the sauce evenly on the top. Repeat layers, ending with cheese. Bake for 25 to 30 minutes or until bubbly.

Nutritional information per serving
*Calories 268, Protein (g) 20, Carbohydrate (g) 34,
Fat (g) 5, Cal. from Fat (%) 18, Saturated Fat (g) 2,
Dietary Fiber (g) 3, Cholesterol (mg) 34, Sodium (mg) 542,
Diabetic Exchanges: 2 very lean meat, 2 starch,
1 vegetable*

DOC'S NOTES:

The bell peppers and tomatoes and chiles are an excellent source of vitamin C. Tomatoes also have lycopene, a cancer fighting antioxidant.

CAREGIVER

Chicken and Black Bean Enchiladas ❄

Adjust the seasoning to your taste for this true Southwestern meal. Freezes well — freeze before baking and add sauce when removed from the freezer and ready to bake.

MAKES 24 ENCHILADAS

2 pounds skinless, boneless chicken breasts,
  cut into cubes
Salt and pepper to taste
1/2 teaspoon minced garlic
1 teaspoon chili powder
1 teaspoon ground cumin
1 (15-ounce) can black beans, drained and rinsed
1 (4-ounce) can chopped green chiles,
  drained, optional
1 cup chopped green onions (scallions)
1 (8-ounce) package shredded reduced-fat
  Monterey Jack cheese
24 (8-inch) flour tortillas
Sauce (recipe follows)

Preheat oven to 350 degrees. In a large skillet coated with nonstick cooking spray over a medium-high heat, cook the chicken, stirring occasionally, until done, about 10 minutes. Season with salt and pepper, garlic, chili powder, and cumin. Add the black beans, green chiles, and green onions, stirring to combine. Remove from the heat. Divide the chicken mixture and cheese evenly among the flour tortillas. Roll up each tortilla tightly and place side by side in a 3-quart casserole. Pour the sauce over the enchiladas. Bake, uncovered, for about 30 minutes.

SAUCE

1/2 cup all-purpose flour
13/4 cups canned fat-free chicken broth
2 cups skim milk
1/2 cup shredded reduced-fat Cheddar cheese
Salt and pepper to taste
1 teaspoon dry mustard
1 tablespoon Worcestershire sauce
1 cup nonfat plain yogurt

In a medium saucepan, place the flour and gradually stir in the chicken broth and milk. Cook, stirring constantly, until the mixture comes to a boil and the sauce thickens. Mix in the cheese, salt and pepper, mustard, and Worcestershire sauce and stir until the cheese melts. Remove from the heat and add the yogurt; do not boil.

Nutritional Information per serving
Calories 225, Protein (g) 20, Carbohydrate (g) 23, Fat (g) 6, Cal. from Fat (%) 24, Saturated Fat (g) 3, Dietary Fiber (g) 3, Cholesterol (mg) 29, Sodium (mg) 278, Diabetic Exchanges: 2 lean meat, 1.5 starch

Seafood and Wild Rice Casserole

An excellent choice! It can be made ahead and reheated.

MAKES 6 TO 8 SERVINGS

1 (6-ounce) package long grain and wild rice mix
1 pound cooked shrimp, peeled
1 pound white crabmeat
1 (10-ounce) package green peas (uncooked)
1 cup chopped celery
1 green bell pepper, cored and chopped
1 onion, chopped
½ cup light mayonnaise
1 teaspoon Worcestershire sauce
Salt and pepper to taste

Preheat oven to 350 degrees. Cook rice mix according to directions on package. Combine rice with all remaining ingredients, tossing carefully. Pour into a 2-quart casserole coated with nonstick cooking spray. Bake for 20 to 30 minutes.

Nutritional information per serving
Calories 287, Protein (g) 29, Carbohydrate (g) 26, Fat (g) 7, Cal. from Fat (%) 21, Saturated Fat (g) 1, Dietary Fiber (g) 3, Cholesterol (mg) 159, Sodium (mg) 833, Diabetic Exchanges: 4 very lean meat, 1.5 starch, 1 vegetable, 0.5 fat

DOC'S NOTES:

This recipe is a good source of protein and fiber.

Turkey Jambalaya ❄

This is a quick and tasty one-dish meal. Jambalaya is a rice mixture combined with seasonings and is a great way to use leftover turkey; you can be a hit twice. Cheat and purchase a roasted chicken to use for the diced turkey.

MAKES 8 TO 10 SERVINGS

1 pound turkey sausage or low-fat sausage

1 large onion, chopped

1 pound fresh mushrooms, sliced

2 (6-ounce) packages long grain and
   wild rice mix

1½ pounds cooked, diced turkey breasts or thighs
   (4 cups)

1 (14-ounce) can artichoke hearts, quartered

½ cup chopped green onions (scallions)

Cut sausage into pieces and brown in large pot coated with nonstick cooking spray. Add onions and mushrooms, cooking until tender. Drain off any excess grease. Add wild rice, seasoning packet and water to sausage mixture and cook according to package directions. Add turkey and artichoke hearts, tossing gently. Top with chopped green onions.

Nutritional information per serving
Calories 366, Protein (g) 36, Carbohydrate (g) 35, Fat (g) 9, Cal. from Fat (%) 23, Saturated Fat (g) 3, Dietary Fiber (g) 3, Cholesterol (mg) 95, Sodium (mg) 979, Diabetic Exchanges: 4 lean meat, 1.5 starch, 2 vegetable

DOC'S NOTES:

Onions are low in calories, while the mushrooms are rich in B Vitamins and minerals. The artichokes are a great source of Vitamin C and dietary fiber.

CAREGIVER

Jumbo Stuffed Shells ❋

A simple favorite that I always double when I prepare. Bring over in foil pans to eat immediately or freeze for a later time.

MAKES 6 TO 8 SERVINGS

1 (12-ounce) package jumbo shells
1½ pounds ground sirloin
2 large egg whites
¼ cup grated Parmesan cheese
¼ cup bread crumbs
1 tablespoon chopped parsley
1 teaspoon dried basil leaves
½ teaspoon dried oregano leaves
Salt and pepper to taste
1 (29-ounce) jar commercial pasta sauce or
   tomato sauce
1 (8-ounce) package shredded part skim
   mozzarella cheese

Preheat oven to 350 degrees. Cook pasta shells according to directions on package omitting oil; drain and set aside. In a skillet, cook sirloin until done. Drain any excess fat. Combine with egg whites, Parmesan cheese, bread crumbs, parsley, basil, oregano, and salt and pepper. Stuff shells with meat filling. Pour half the pasta sauce in a 2-quart baking dish. Arrange stuffed shells on top and cover with remaining sauce. Bake for 20 minutes. Sprinkle with mozzarella cheese and continue baking for 10 minutes longer.

Nutritional information per serving
Calories 478, Protein (g) 33, Carbohydrate (g) 47, Fat (g) 17, Cal. from Fat (%) 32, Saturated Fat (g) 7, Dietary Fiber (g) 3, Cholesterol (mg) 68, Sodium (mg) 787, Diabetic Exchanges: 3.5 lean meat, 2.5 starch, 2 vegetable, 1 fat

DOC'S NOTES:

Everyone seems to enjoy ground beef recipes, and sirloin is a lean cut of beef.

CAREGIVER

Pasta Salad 🥕

An outstanding pasta salad packed full of great ingredients with a wonderful light dressing.

MAKES 10 SERVINGS

2 cups snow peas
1 bunch broccoli, flowerets only
1 (12-ounce) package tri-colored pasta shells
1 (6-ounce) package tri-colored stuffed tortellini
1/2 pound fresh mushrooms, cut in half
1 cup cherry tomatoes, cut in half
1 red bell pepper, cored and cut into strips
1/3 cup grated Romano cheese

Cook snow peas and broccoli in the microwave until crisp tender. Drain and set aside. Cook pasta shells and tortellini according to directions on package omitting salt and oil. Drain and set aside. Combine all ingredients in a large bowl. Toss with Dressing (recipe follows).

DRESSING

1 bunch green onions (scallions), chopped
1/2 cup red wine vinegar
1/3 cup olive oil
2 tablespoons chopped parsley
3 cloves garlic, minced
2 teaspoons dried basil leaves
1 teaspoon dried dill weed leaves
1/2 teaspoon dried oregano leaves
Salt and pepper to taste
1/2 teaspoon sugar
1 1/2 teaspoons Dijon mustard

Combine all ingredients together, mixing well. Pour over pasta salad and refrigerate.

Nutritional information per serving
Calories 283, Protein (g) 10, Carbohydrate (g) 40, Fat (g) 10, Cal. from Fat (%) 31, Saturated Fat (g) 2, Dietary Fiber (g) 4, Cholesterol (mg) 13, Sodium (mg) 334, Diabetic Exchanges: 2 starch, 2 vegetable, 1.5 fat

DOC'S NOTES:

Includes broccoli, a cruciferous vegetable with Vitamins A, B, and C.

Shrimp-Rice Casserole ❄

The hint of cheese and salsa makes this an outstanding quick shrimp and rice dish. Adjust the seasoning to how well you can tolerate them.

MAKES 6 SERVINGS

1 onion, chopped

1 teaspoon minced garlic

½ cup chopped red or green bell pepper

1½ pounds medium shrimp, peeled

1 (8-ounce) can mushroom stems and
   pieces, drained

1½ cups shredded reduced-fat Cheddar cheese

⅓ cup salsa

1 tablespoon Worcestershire sauce

½ cup evaporated skimmed milk

1 bunch green onions (scallions),
   chopped, optional

2 tablespoons canned diced green chiles,
   drained, optional

3 cups cooked white or brown rice

In a large skillet coated with nonstick cooking spray, sauté the onion, garlic, pepper, shrimp, and mushrooms over medium-high heat for about 5 to 7 minutes. Add the cheese, salsa, Worcestershire sauce, evaporated milk, green onions, and green chiles. Stir in the rice and cook until the cheese is melted and well combined.

Nutritional information per serving

Calories 317, Protein (g) 31, Carbohydrate (g) 31, Fat (g) 6, Cal. from Fat (%) 18, Saturated Fat (g) 4, Dietary Fiber (g) 2, Cholesterol (mg) 177, Sodium (mg) 648, Diabetic Exchanges: 3.5 very lean meat, 1.5 starch, 1 vegetable

DOC'S NOTES:

Buy peeled shrimp or have a friend peel them for you. You do not want to prick your finger on a shrimp shell while your white blood cell count is low. Wonderful dish!

Pretzel Strawberry Gelatin 🥕

This delicious recipe will even pass for dessert. A great choice!

MAKES 16 SERVINGS

4 tablespoons margarine, melted

2 tablespoons light brown sugar

2 cups crushed pretzels

1 (6-ounce) package strawberry gelatin

2 cups boiling water

3 cups sliced fresh strawberries

4 ounces fat-free cream cheese

½ cup sugar

1 (1.3-ounce) envelope dry whipped topping mix

½ cup skim milk

Preheat oven to 350 degrees. Combine margarine, brown sugar and pretzels and press into a 13×9×2-inch baking pan. Bake for 10 minutes; cool. Meanwhile dissolve strawberry gelatin in boiling water, stirring until dissolved. Add sliced strawberries. Cool in refrigerator until gelatin begins to set. In mixer, beat cream cheese with sugar. Prepare whipped topping according to directions on package substituting skim milk. Fold into cream cheese mixture. Spread over cooled crust. Pour semi-firm gelatin mixture over cream cheese layer. Refrigerate until congealed.

Nutritional information per serving
Calories 163, Protein (g) 3, Carbohydrate (g) 30, Fat (g) 4, Cal. from Fat (%) 20, Saturated Fat (g) 1, Dietary Fiber (g) 1, Cholesterol (mg) 1, Sodium (mg) 258, Diabetic Exchanges: 0.5 starch, 1.5 other carb., 0.5 fat

DOC'S NOTES:

Gelatin is great for your nails which are sometimes weakened by chemotherapy. This is also a great source of Vitamin C and potassium.

Tropical Pizza 🥕

Have fun with this pizza by adding your favorite fruit and creating it in the pattern of your choice. With fresh fruit in season, this picture perfect dessert is even more nutritious.

MAKES 12 SERVINGS

1 (18-ounce) roll refrigerated ready to slice
   sugar cookie dough
1/3 cup sugar
1 (8-ounce) package fat-free cream cheese
1 teaspoon coconut extract
1 1/2 teaspoons grated orange rind
1 cup frozen fat-free whipped topping, thawed
1 (26-ounce) jar mango slices, drained
1 (16-ounce) can pineapple slices, drained
1 (11-ounce) can mandarin orange
   slices, drained
1/4 cup apricot preserves
1 tablespoon orange liqueur, optional
2 tablespoons coconut, toasted, optional

Preheat oven to 350 degrees. Press the cookie dough into a 12 to 14-inch pizza pan coated with nonstick cooking spray. Bake for 12 minutes and cool completely. In a mixing bowl, blend together sugar, cream cheese, and coconut extract until well mixed. Stir in the orange rind and whipped topping, mixing until smooth. Spread the cream cheese mixture on top of the cooled crust. Arrange the mango slices around the edge of the iced pizza. Next, arrange a row of the pineapple slices around the inside of the mango slices. Arrange the mandarin orange slices to fill the center of the pizza. In a small saucepan or in the microwave, heat the apricot preserves and orange liqueur just until melted. Spoon the glaze over the fruit. Sprinkle with the toasted coconut if desired. Refrigerate until serving.

Nutritional information per serving
Calories 277, Protein (g) 5, Carbohydrate (g) 51, Fat (g) 6, Cal. from Fat (%) 20, Saturated Fat (g) 2, Dietary Fiber (g) 1, Cholesterol (mg) 5, Sodium (mg) 249, Diabetic Exchanges: 1 starch, 1 fruit, 1.5 other carb., 1 fat

DOC'S NOTES:

One slice per day will aid in your constipation problem plus provide Vitamin C. Vitamins C and E, along with beta carotene are antioxidant vitamins. The antioxidants seem to neutralize a class of atomic particles known as "free radicals." The free radicals combine with other compounds, creating a chain reaction and, over the course of time, will damage cell walls and structure within the cells.

CAREGIVER

Chocolate Layered Dessert 🥕

Easy, a favorite, and will satisfy that sweet tooth when you want dessert.

MAKES 16 SERVINGS

CRUST

1 cup flour
7 tablespoons margarine
1/2 cup chopped pecans

Preheat oven to 350 degrees. Mix all ingredients and press into an ungreased 13×9×2-inch pan. Bake for 20 minutes. Cool and then top with Cream Cheese Layer (recipe follows). Refrigerate until serving.

CREAM CHEESE LAYER

3/4 cup frozen fat-free whipped topping
1 (8-ounce) package fat-free cream cheese
2/3 cup powdered sugar

Combine ingredients in mixer and beat only until well blended. Spread on top of first layer. Top with Pudding Layer (recipe follows).

PUDDING LAYER

1 (4-serving) package instant vanilla pudding
1 (4-serving) package instant chocolate pudding
3 cups skim milk
1 teaspoon vanilla extract
1 1/4 cups frozen fat-free whipped topping, thawed

Mix pudding with milk and beat according to directions on package. After thickened, add vanilla. Spread on top of Cream Cheese Layer. Cover dessert with whipped topping.

Nutritional information per serving

Calories 207, Protein (g) 5, Carbohydrate (g) 29, Fat (g) 8, Cal. from Fat (%) 34, Saturated Fat (g) 1, Dietary Fiber (g) 1, Cholesterol (mg) 2, Sodium (mg) 333, Diabetic Exchanges: 0.5 starch, 1.5 other carb., 1.5 fat

DOC'S NOTES:

It is hard to believe this is low fat. Vanilla nutritional energy drink supplement can be substituted for the skim milk to turn this into a high calorie dessert. This is an easily tolerated choice.

Sweet Potato Pound Cake 🥕 ❄️

The orange glaze over the spicy moist cake will make this a sensational choice for dessert. Sweet potatoes are rich in beta carotene, and Vitamins C and E.

MAKES 16 SERVINGS

½ cup margarine

1 cup sugar

1 large egg

3 large egg whites

2 (15-ounce) cans sweet potatoes (yams), drained and mashed (about 2 cups)

1 teaspoon vanilla extract

2½ cups all-purpose flour

1 teaspoon baking powder

1 teaspoon baking soda

1 teaspoon ground cinnamon

½ teaspoon ground nutmeg

1 teaspoon grated orange rind

⅓ cup flaked coconut

½ cup coarsely chopped walnuts, optional

2-3 tablespoons orange juice

1 cup confectioners' sugar

Preheat oven to 350 degrees. In a mixing bowl, beat together margarine and sugar until blended. Add egg and egg whites, one at a time, beating well after each addition. Mix in sweet potatoes and vanilla. In another bowl, mix together flour, baking powder, baking soda, cinnamon, nutmeg, and orange rind. Gradually spoon flour mixture into creamed mixture, beating well after each addition. Stir in coconut and walnuts. Pour batter into a 10-inch Bundt pan coated with nonstick cooking spray. Bake 45 to 50 minutes or until a wooden pick inserted in center of cake comes out clean. Cool in pan for 10 minutes; invert onto a serving plate. In a small bowl, mix together orange juice and confectioners' sugar to make a glaze. Spoon glaze over cake.

Nutritional information per serving
Calories 249, Protein (g) 4, Carbohydrate (g) 44, Fat (g) 7, Cal. from Fat (%) 24, Saturated Fat (g) 2, Dietary Fiber (g) 1, Cholesterol (mg) 13, Sodium (mg) 219, Diabetic Exchanges: 1.5 starch, 1.5 other carb., 1 fat

DOC'S NOTES:

Sweet potatoes are rich in beta-carotene, and important nutrients making this a dessert with added nutrition.

CAREGIVER

Healthy Eating
Post Treatment

+ Do I have to follow a special diet?
+ Is it okay to eat raw fruits and vegetables?
+ Are there any foods that decrease my risk of cancer?
+ What is the most important food to decrease for healthy living — you're right — **FAT**!
+ What about carcinogens — a cancer producing substance?

Once your treatments are over, you will hopefully start to feel better and will be eager to try new foods. Your taste buds are alert and again ready to be stimulated. You do not have to worry about your blood count being low or your mouth being sore. Hopefully, your bowel habits have normalized. It is fine to eat raw fruits and vegetables.

Salt-cured and pickled foods contain natural carcinogens that may increase your risk of developing stomach and esophageal cancers. Nitrates and nitrites, used to preserve meats, can enhance the formation of nitrosoamine, another carcinogen. Smoked foods can absorb carcinogens out of the smoke.

The good foods, such as whole grains, legumes, fruits, and vegetables, will decrease your risk of cancer. These foods all contain dietary fiber, which is thought to protect against colon cancer. Diets high in fruits and vegetables are believed to protect against bladder, prostate, stomach, esophageal, and lung cancer. Please do not forget smoking is the very worst carcinogen around. Smoking is responsible for lung, bladder, esophageal, and head and neck cancer. Eat healthy, but PLEASE DO NOT SMOKE. Cruciferous vegetables (kale, cauliflower, broccoli) may also reduce your risk of cancer. Foods rich in vitamin C can protect against cancers of the mouth, esophagus, pancreas, and stomach.

Vitamins A and E may help protect against certain cancers by acting as antioxidants, and in the case of vitamin E, by inhibiting the conversion of nitrites into nitrosamines. Green tea may protect against some cancers by stimulating the activity of antioxidant and detoxifying enzymes.

Also note that a diet that reduces your risk of developing cancer can also reduce your risk of developing heart disease. It can also decrease your risk of developing diverticulitis and irritable bowel syndrome, both of which have been linked to a diet low in fiber.

There are more studies on fat than on any dietary risk factor. There is good evidence that fat increases your risk of developing cancer, especially cancer of the prostate, colon, breast, ovary, endometrium, and pancreas. The National Cancer Institute (NCI) and the American Cancer Society both recommend that you limit your fat intake to 30% or less of the calories you consume.

How can you cut down on fat:
(1) Eat skinless chicken breasts.
(2) Select meat with loin or round in the name—ground sirloin.
(3) Replace meat with beans, fish or chicken.
(4) Replace whole milk with nonfat or 1% milk.
(5) Replace ice cream with sherbet or frozen yogurt or use low-fat products.
(6) Substitute croissants and breakfast bars with bagels, English muffins, whole grain bread, pita bread or corn tortillas.
(7) Be conscious of your choice of food.

Remember you do not have to deprive yourself forever of the foods you love. If you overdo it one day, make allowances the next day or two. The method of healthy eating Monday through Friday and splurging on the weekends sometimes works well for people. It is important that you find the balance of what works best for you. Your goal is a long term healthy lifestyle. With all these tasty recipes, you will find that your diet will not be different than the next person as it is the approach in preparation of these recipes that has changed. Enjoy eating and staying healthy.

Dietary Suggestions for A Healthy Diet
◆ Keep your total fat intake at or below 30% of your total calories, and limit your intake of saturated fats—which contribute to high blood cholesterol levels—to no more than 10% of your total calories.
◆ Limit your intake of dietary cholesterol to no more than 300 milligrams per day.
◆ Get at least 55% of your total daily calories from carbohydrates, preferably complex carbohydrates—the starches in grains, legumes, vegetables, and some fruits. These foods can also provide you with the 20 to 30 grams of dietary fiber that is recommended daily, as well as vitamins and minerals.

- ✦ Protein should make up only about 12 to 15% of your daily calories—the protein should come from low-fat sources.
- ✦ Avoid too much sugar; it contributes to tooth decay, and many foods high in sugar are also high in fat.
- ✦ Try to limit your sodium to no more than 2400 milligrams per day, the equivalent of a little more than a teaspoon of salt.
- ✦ Maintain an adequate intake of vitamins and minerals—particularly of iron and calcium.
- ✦ If you drink alcohol, do so in moderation—no more than one ounce of alcohol a day, if at all.

Guidelines To Prevent Cancer
- ✦ Reduce saturated fat intake.
- ✦ Increase consumption of fruits and vegetables, especially cruciferous.
- ✦ Reduce consumption of salt-cured and smoked foods.
- ✦ Continue efforts to minimize contamination of foods with carcinogens from any source.
- ✦ Consume alcohol in moderation, if at all.
- ✦ Do not smoke.
- ✦ Exercise.

Oatmeal Pancakes 🥕 ❄️

These hearty whole grain pancakes are wonderful. Try cutting up bananas in the batter or top with sliced fruit instead of syrup.

MAKES ABOUT **10** PANCAKES

1/2 cup whole wheat flour
1 teaspoon baking powder
1 tablespoon light brown sugar
1/2 teaspoon ground cinnamon
1 1/2 cups cooked oatmeal
3/4 cup skim milk
1 tablespoon canola oil
1 large egg

Mix together flour, baking powder, sugar, and cinnamon. Stir into oatmeal. Mix milk, oil, and egg together and add to batter. Cook pancakes on a heated skillet coated with nonstick cooking spray.

Nutritional information per serving
Calories 74, Protein (g) 3, Carbohydrate (g) 11, Fat (g) 2, Cal. from Fat (%) 28, Saturated Fat (g) 0, Dietary Fiber (g) 1, Cholesterol (mg) 22, Sodium (mg) 66, Diabetic Exchanges: 0.5 starch, 0.5 fat

DOC'S NOTES:

A great way to include fiber in your meal. Top with blueberries for a big dose of antioxidants.

Beefy Vegetable Soup ❄

This makes a huge pot of soup. Freeze in containers and have dinner in only minutes. Remember, you can always add your favorite fresh or frozen vegetables to the pot. Great way to clean out the refrigerator. For a quick version, use cans of beef broth.

MAKES SIXTEEN (1-CUP) SERVINGS

2 pounds extra-lean stewing beef, cubed
1 pound cross-cut beef shank, cubed
6 quarts water
Salt and pepper to taste
1 large onion, chopped
1 cup chopped celery
1 (16-ounce) package frozen corn
1 (16-ounce) package frozen cut green beans
1 (16-ounce) package baby carrots
2 cups shredded cabbage
2 (28-ounce) cans no-salt added whole tomatoes, with their juice
2 bay leaves
1 (8-ounce) package small shell pasta

In a very large pot, place the stewing beef, beef shank, and 6 quarts of water. Season with salt and pepper. Bring to a boil and boil 1 to 1½ hours over medium heat. Add the onion, celery, corn, green beans, carrots, cabbage, tomatoes, and bay leaves. Continue cooking for 1 hour. Add the pasta and cook until the pasta is done and meat is tender, about 10 to 15 minutes. Season to taste and remove the bay leaves before serving. Add more water or beef broth if soup gets too thick.

Nutritional information per serving

Calories 237, Protein (g) 24, Carbohydrate (g) 27, Fat (g) 4, Cal. from Fat (%) 15, Saturated Fat (g) 1, Dietary Fiber (g) 4, Cholesterol (mg) 46, Sodium (mg) 75, Diabetic Exchanges: 2.5 very lean meat, 1 starch, 3 vegetable

DOC'S NOTES:

High fiber content with a great source of Vitamins A and C. Cabbage is a cruciferous vegetable.

Couscous Salad

Couscous only takes minutes to prepare and this wonderful combination of cranberries, snow peas, and peanuts makes this recipe a wonderful choice.

MAKES 8 TO 10 SERVINGS

1 teaspoon minced garlic, divided

4 tablespoons lemon juice, divided

2 1/2 cups canned fat-free chicken broth

1 1/2 cups couscous

1/3 cup chopped fresh parsley

1 (10-ounce) package snow peas, cooked crisp tender according to directions

5 green onions (scallions), chopped

1/2 cup peanuts

1/2 cup dried cranberries

2 tablespoons olive oil

Dash of hot pepper sauce

In a pot coated with nonstick cooking spray, sauté 1/2 teaspoon garlic and add 1 tablespoon lemon juice and chicken broth. Bring to a full boil and add couscous, cover pot and remove from heat. Let sit for 5 minutes, fluff with a fork and add parsley. Set aside to cool. When cool, add snow peas, green onions, peanuts, and cranberries. For dressing, mix together remaining 1/2 teaspoon minced garlic and 3 tablespoons lemon juice, oil, and hot sauce. Toss the dressing with the couscous mixture.

Nutritional information per serving

Calories 204, Protein (g) 7, Carbohydrate (g) 30, Fat (g) 7, Cal. from Fat (%) 29, Saturated Fat (g) 1, Dietary Fiber (g) 4, Cholesterol (mg) 0, Sodium (mg) 162, Diabetic Exchanges: 1.5 starch, 0.5 fruit, 1 fat

DOC'S NOTES:

A high fiber recipe with the ingredients providing calcium and vitamin C.

Paella Salad

This attractive salad of many colors and textures will convince even the heartiest eaters that a salad can make a satisfying meal. The shrimp may be left out.

MAKES 6 SERVINGS

2 (5-ounce) packages saffron yellow rice

1/4 cup balsamic vinegar

1/4 cup lemon juice

1 tablespoon olive oil

1 teaspoon dried basil leaves

1/8 teaspoon black pepper

Dash of cayenne pepper

1 pound medium shrimp, peeled and cooked

1 (14-ounce) can quartered artichoke
  hearts, drained

3/4 cup chopped green bell pepper

1 cup frozen green peas, thawed

1 cup chopped tomato

1 (2-ounce) jar diced pimentos, drained

1/2 cup chopped red onion

2 ounces chopped prosciutto, optional

Prepare the rice according to package directions, omitting any oil and salt. Set aside. In a small bowl, mix together the vinegar, lemon juice, oil, basil, black pepper, and cayenne pepper; set dressing aside. In a large bowl, combine the cooked rice with the shrimp, artichoke hearts, green pepper, peas, tomato, pimentos, red onion, and prosciutto, mixing well. Pour the dressing over the rice mixture, tossing to coat. Cover and refrigerate at least 2 hours before serving.

Nutritional information per serving

Calories 290, Protein (g) 17, Carbohydrate (g) 50, Fat (g) 3, Cal. from Fat (%) 9, Saturated Fat (g) 1, Dietary Fiber (g) 3, Cholesterol (mg) 90, Sodium (mg) 871, Diabetic Exchanges: 1.5 very lean meat, 3 starch, 1 vegetable

DOC'S NOTES:

Low in fat and high in fiber.

Seven-Layer Salad

A fantastic make-ahead layered salad with a divine dressing.

MAKES 8 TO 10 SERVINGS

1/2 cup nonfat plain yogurt

1/2 cup buttermilk

1/2 cup crumbled feta cheese (about 2 ounces)

1 teaspoon sugar

1/4 teaspoon dried dill weed leaves

1/2 teaspoon dried basil leaves

1/8 teaspoon ground white pepper

1 (9-ounce) package spinach tortellini

6 cups torn fresh spinach leaves

1/2 pound fresh mushrooms, sliced

2 Roma (plum) tomatoes, chopped

4 green onions (scallions), chopped

2 1/2 ounces sliced Canadian bacon, pan-cooked and cut into pieces, optional

In a food processor, blend the yogurt, buttermilk, feta cheese, sugar, dill weed, basil, and pepper until smooth to make a dressing. Chill. Cook the tortellini according to package directions, omitting any oil and salt. Drain and rinse in cold water. In a 3-quart oblong dish, layer the spinach leaves, tortellini, mushrooms, tomatoes, and green onions. Pour the dressing over the salad and sprinkle with the bacon. Cover and refrigerate at least 2 hours or overnight to blend the flavors until serving time.

Nutritional information per serving

Calories 96, Protein (g) 6, Carbohydrate (g) 10, Fat (g) 4, Cal. from Fat (%) 35, Saturated Fat (g) 2, Dietary Fiber (g) 1, Cholesterol (mg) 40, Sodium (mg) 176, Diabetic Exchanges: 1 lean meat, 0.5 starch

DOC'S NOTES:

Spinach is high in iron, Vitamin A and calcium. The tomatoes provide Vitamins A and C.

Sweet and Sour Broccoli Salad 🥕

This salad will receive rave reviews.

MAKES 6 SERVINGS

4 cups broccoli florets, cut in small pieces
1/2 cup chopped green onions (scallions)
2 cups red or green grapes, or combination
1 head red tip lettuce, torn into pieces
1 tablespoon margarine
1/4 cup slivered almonds
1/2 cup red wine vinegar
1/4 cup sugar
2 tablespoons reduced-sodium soy sauce
1 tablespoon olive oil

In a large bowl, combine the broccoli, green onions, grapes, and lettuce; set aside. In a small skillet coated with nonstick cooking spray, melt the margarine. Add the almonds and sauté until light brown; set aside. In a small bowl, whisk together the red wine vinegar, sugar, soy sauce, and olive oil. Pour over the broccoli mixture and toss. Stir in the browned almonds.

Nutritional information per serving
Calories 165, Protein (g) 4, Carbohydrate (g) 23, Fat (g) 8, Cal. from Fat (%) 39, Saturated Fat (g) 1, Dietary Fiber (g) 3, Cholesterol (mg) 0, Sodium (mg) 242, Diabetic Exchanges: 0.5 fruit, 1 vegetable, 0.5 other carb., 1.5 fat

DOC'S NOTES:

Broccoli is in the cruciferous family. Broccoli contains indoles which are effective in protecting against certain forms of cancer. It has a rich supply of vitamins and minerals.

Caesar Salad

You will not miss the "real thing" with this duplication. For a light dinner, top with grilled chicken.

MAKES 4 SERVINGS

2 tablespoons grated Parmesan cheese

2 tablespoons water

2 tablespoons red wine vinegar

1 teaspoon Worcestershire sauce

1 tablespoon olive oil

1 clove garlic

1/4 teaspoon dry mustard

1 large bunch romaine lettuce, cleaned and torn into pieces

1/3 cup croutons, optional

Combine all ingredients except lettuce and croutons in a food processor and blend until smooth. Pour over lettuce, tossing well. Top with croutons, if desired.

Nutritional information per serving

Calories 63, Protein (g) 3, Carbohydrate (g) 3, Fat (g) 5, Cal. from Fat (%) 61, Saturated Fat (g) 1, Dietary Fiber (g) 2, Cholesterol (mg) 3, Sodium (mg) 82, Diabetic Exchanges: 1 vegetable, 1 fat

DOC'S NOTES:

Romaine lettuce is a little more nutritious than iceberg. Great source of Vitamin A, beta carotene, Vitamin C, and folacin.

Raspberry Spinach Salad 🥕

This salad is truly outstanding. Toss with toasted pine nuts for that extra special touch. For a change, use a variety of lettuce instead of spinach.

MAKES 8 SERVINGS

3 tablespoons raspberry vinegar

3 tablespoons seedless raspberry jam

¼ cup canola oil

8 cups fresh spinach, rinsed, stemmed, and torn into pieces

1 cup fresh raspberries or sliced strawberries

3 kiwis, peeled and sliced

Combine vinegar and jam in a food processor or blender. With processor running, add oil in a thin stream, blending well. In a large bowl, carefully toss spinach, raspberries, and kiwis with dressing. Serve immediately.

Nutritional information per serving

Calories 115, Protein (g) 1, Carbohydrate (g) 13, Fat (g) 7, Cal. from Fat (%) 53, Saturated Fat (g) 1, Dietary Fiber (g) 3, Cholesterol (mg) 0, Sodium (mg) 26, Diabetic Exchanges: 0.5 fruit, 0.5 other carb., 1.5 fat

DOC'S NOTES:

Get in the habit of adding fruit of your choice to your salad.

Tropical Green Salad 🥕

Depending on the time of year, use available fruit instead of nectarines to create this tropical paradise salad. Avocado and olive oil are great choices for monounsaturated fat, which has been cited as preventative for cancer.

MAKES 8 SERVINGS

2 cups sugar snap peas
6 cups torn assorted lettuce
1 avocado, pitted and cut into 1-inch cubes
3 nectarines, sliced
1/4 cup sunflower seeds
1/2 cup thinly sliced red onion
1/4 cup lime juice
2 tablespoons olive oil
3 tablespoons honey

Cook the sugar snap peas in a covered microwave dish in a small amount of water, about 4 minutes or until crisp tender. Drain, rinse with cold water, and set aside. In a large bowl, combine the cooked snap peas, lettuce, avocado, nectarines, sunflower seeds, and onion. In a small bowl, whisk together the lime juice, oil, and honey. Toss dressing with salad mixture.

Nutritional information per serving
Calories 165, Protein (g) 3, Carbohydrate (g) 20, Fat (g) 9, Cal. from Fat (%) 47, Saturated Fat (g) 1, Dietary Fiber (g) 5, Cholesterol (mg) 0, Sodium (mg) 11, Diabetic Exchanges: 0.5 fruit, 1 vegetable, 0.5 other carb., 2 fat

DOC'S NOTES:

Excellent source of vitamins, calcium and fiber.

Spinach Rice with Feta 🥕

Adjust the onion and mushrooms to your preferences. Spinach and feta compliment each other, however, the cheese of choice can be used or even delete cheese.

MAKES 6 SERVINGS

1 cup dry brown rice

2¼ cups canned fat-free chicken broth

1 medium onion, chopped

½ pound sliced mushrooms

½ teaspoon minced garlic

1 tablespoon lemon juice

1 teaspoon dried oregano leaves

1 (10-ounce) bag fresh spinach leaves, stemmed

½ cup crumbled feta cheese

In a saucepan, combine rice and broth. Bring to a boil, stir, and reduce heat. Cover and simmer for 35 to 45 minutes or until rice is tender. Meanwhile, in a large skillet coated with nonstick cooking spray, sauté the onion, mushrooms, and garlic until tender. Stir in lemon juice and oregano. Add spinach, cooking only until wilted. Toss cooked rice with spinach mixture. Sprinkle with cheese and serve.

Nutritional information per serving

Calories 184, Protein (g) 8, Carbohydrate (g) 31, Fat (g) 4, Cal. from Fat (%) 18, Saturated Fat (g) 2, Dietary Fiber (g) 3, Cholesterol (mg) 11, Sodium (mg) 414, Diabetic Exchanges: 1.5 starch, 1 vegetable, 0.5 fat

DOC'S NOTES:

Spinach is a wonderful source of minerals.

Fried Rice Stir-Fry 🥕

Turn that leftover rice into a light veggie meal. The eggs give the dish protein. If you have sesame oil, you may add a tablespoon instead of the last tablespoon peanut oil.

MAKES 6 SERVINGS

2 large eggs
2 tablespoons peanut oil, divided
1 onion, chopped
1 tablespoon minced garlic
¼ cup reduced sodium soy sauce
4 cups cooked white or brown rice
1 bunch green onions (scallions), chopped
⅓ cup sliced water chestnuts
1 cup frozen green peas

Coat a 12-inch nonstick skillet with nonstick cooking spray and set it over medium heat. Beat the eggs lightly, pour them into the skillet, and cook without stirring until they are almost dry. When the eggs are ready, remove them to a plate and cut into strips; set aside. In the same skillet, heat 1 tablespoon oil and sauté the onion and garlic until tender. Add the soy sauce, rice, and remaining 1 tablespoon oil, stirring until well heated. Add the green onions, water chestnuts, and peas, stir frying until well heated. Gently mix in the egg strips and serve.

Nutritional information per serving

Calories 247, Protein (g) 8, Carbohydrate (g) 39, Fat (g) 7, Cal. from Fat (%) 24, Saturated Fat (g) 1, Dietary Fiber (g) 3, Cholesterol (mg) 71, Sodium (mg) 453, Diabetic Exchanges: 2 starch, 2 vegetable, 1 fat

DOC'S NOTE:

This recipe is packed with vitamins A and C and calcium. Brown rice is a good source of vitamin E and fiber.

Curried Rice and Sweet Potatoes 🥕

If you enjoy curry, this team of rice and sweet potatoes makes a great side dish. By including apples, raisins, and peas you have a variety of nutrients in one dish.

MAKES 6 SERVINGS

¹⁄₂ cup chopped onion
¹⁄₂ teaspoon minced garlic
1 cup dry rice
2 cups water
2 cups peeled and diced sweet potatoes (yams)
1 cup peeled and chopped Granny Smith apple
1 cup frozen peas
¹⁄₃ cup golden raisins
¹⁄₂ cup walnuts, toasted
1 teaspoon curry powder
Salt to taste

In a pot coated with nonstick cooking spray, sauté the onion and garlic until tender. Add the rice, water, and sweet potatoes; bring to a boil. Cover, reduce heat, and simmer 15 minutes or until the liquid is absorbed. Carefully stir in the apple, peas, raisins, walnuts, curry, and salt.

Nutritional information per serving

Calories 277, Protein (g) 6, Carbohydrate (g) 51, Fat (g) 6, Cal. from Fat (%) 19, Saturated Fat (g) 1, Dietary Fiber (g) 5, Cholesterol (mg) 0, Sodium (mg) 36, Diabetic Exchanges: 2.5 starch, 1 fruit, 1 fat

DOC'S NOTES:

Packed with tons of vitamins and fiber.

Easy Broccoli Potato Bake 🥕 ❄️

By including broccoli in this easy, fabulous potato dish, you are getting in your veggies. The broccoli can be omitted for a plain potato bake.

MAKES 8 TO 10 SERVINGS

2 (10-ounce) packages frozen broccoli, thawed
1 (32-ounce) bag frozen hash brown potatoes
2 cups shredded reduced-fat sharp
   Cheddar cheese
1 (16-ounce) container low-fat cottage cheese
2 cups nonfat plain yogurt
Salt and pepper to taste
Paprika

Preheat oven to 350 degrees. In a 3-quart casserole dish coated with nonstick cooking spray, combine all ingredients except paprika, mixing well. Sprinkle with paprika. Bake 1 hour 15 minutes to 1 hour 30 minutes or until casserole is bubbly.

Nutritional information per serving

Calories 214, Protein (g) 18, Carbohydrate (g) 25, Fat (g) 5, Cal. from Fat (%) 22, Saturated Fat (g) 3, Dietary Fiber (g) 3, Cholesterol (mg) 19, Sodium (mg) 361, Diabetic Exchanges: 1.5 lean meat, 1 starch, 0.5 skim milk, 1 vegetable

DOC'S NOTES:

Another way to get cruciferous vegetables in your diet.

Cauliflower
Supreme

Purchase cauliflower and broccoli flowerets for an easy combo.

MAKES 4 SERVINGS

1 head cauliflower, cut into flowerets
1/3 cup water
1/2 cup nonfat plain yogurt
1/2 cup shredded reduced fat sharp
  Cheddar cheese
1/2 teaspoon dry mustard
Dash of cayenne pepper
Salt and pepper to taste

Preheat oven to 400 degrees. Cook cauliflower in 1/3 cup water, covered, in microwave for 8 minutes or until crisp tender. Drain and transfer to a baking dish coated with nonstick cooking spray. Combine yogurt with remaining ingredients and spread over cauliflower. Bake, uncovered, for 8 to 10 minutes or until lightly browned.

Nutritional information per serving

Calories 96, Protein (g) 9, Carbohydrate (g) 10, Fat (g) 3, Cal. from Fat (%) 25, Saturated Fat (g) 2, Dietary Fiber (g) 3, Cholesterol (mg) 8, Sodium (mg) 158, Diabetic Exchanges: 1 lean meat, 2 vegetable

DOC'S NOTES:

Cauliflower is a member of the cruciferous family. Like broccoli, members of this family have been associated with reducing the risk of cancer.

Pesto Pasta 🥕

This easily prepared pesto tossed with pasta turns a simple dish into a powerhouse of taste. Add some sautéed tomatoes and fresh baby spinach for a real health enhancing Italian dish.

MAKES 4 TO 6 SERVINGS

1/4 cup blanched almonds
1 cup firmly packed fresh basil leaves
4 cloves garlic
3 tablespoons olive oil
3 tablespoons grated Parmesan cheese
1/4 cup canned fat-free chicken broth
Salt and pepper to taste
1 (12-ounce) package angel hair pasta

Place the almonds in a food processor and process until finely chopped; set aside. Add the basil and garlic to the food processor until coarsely chopped. Add the oil, cheese, broth, and salt and pepper. Process until finely minced. Add the reserved almonds; process until mixed. Add more broth if needed to thin. Cook the pasta according to package directions; drain and mix with pesto.

Nutritional information per serving
Calories 326, Protein (g) 10, Carbohydrate (g) 45, Fat (g) 12, Cal. from Fat (%) 33, Saturated Fat (g) 2, Dietary Fiber (g) 2, Cholesterol (mg) 3, Sodium (mg) 89, Diabetic Exchanges: 3 starch, 2 fat

DOC'S NOTES:

If you do not have almonds, try toasted pecans.

Squash and Tomato Casserole 🥕 ❄️

When squash is in season, this tasty recipe will enhance any dinner. Even if you're not a squash fan, give this recipe a try as it's very good.

MAKES 6 TO 8 SERVINGS

2 pounds yellow squash, sliced

1 onion, finely minced

1 teaspoon minced garlic

Salt and pepper to taste

4 slices reduced-fat American cheese

1 (16-ounce) can diced tomatoes, drained, or
   1 cup chopped fresh tomatoes

Preheat oven to 350 degrees. In a large skillet coated with nonstick cooking spray, sauté squash, onion, garlic, and salt and pepper, stirring, about 10 minutes or until veggies are tender. Remove from heat, drain excess liquid. Add cheese, stirring until cheese melts. Pour mixture into an 8-inch square casserole. Sprinkle tomatoes over squash. Bake for 20 to 25 minutes.

Nutritional information per serving

Calories 60, Protein (g) 5, Carbohydrate (g) 10, Fat (g) 1, Cal. from Fat (%) 14, Saturated Fat (g) 1, Dietary Fiber (g) 3, Cholesterol (mg) 4, Sodium (mg) 237, Diabetic Exchanges: 0.5 lean meat, 2 vegetable

DOC'S NOTES:

The squash and tomatoes make this an excellent source of Vitamin A.

Yam Cornbread Stuffing 🥕 ❄️

By adding yams to your traditional stuffing, you add nutrition.

MAKES 10 SERVINGS

2 cups chopped and peeled raw sweet
   potatoes (yams)
1 cup chopped onion
1 cup chopped celery
2 tablespoons margarine
1/4 cup chopped parsley
1 teaspoon ground ginger
5 cups crumbled cornbread
1/4 cup chopped pecans
Chicken broth or vegetable broth

Preheat oven to 375 degrees. In a large skillet, cook sweet potatoes, onion, and celery in margarine for 5 to 7 minutes or until just tender. Spoon mixture into a large mixing bowl. Stir in parsley and ginger. Add cornbread and pecans. Toss gently to coat. Add enough chicken broth to moisten. Place stuffing in a casserole. Bake, uncovered, for 45 minutes or until heated through.

Nutritional information per serving
Calories 157, Protein (g) 3, Carbohydrate (g) 21, Fat (g) 7, Cal. from Fat (%) 40, Saturated Fat (g) 1, Dietary Fiber (g) 3, Cholesterol (mg) 12, Sodium (mg) 228, Diabetic Exchanges: 1.5 starch, 1 fat

DOC'S NOTES:

Sweet potatoes are one of the most nutritious foods in the vegetable kingdom. A 5-inch sweet potato contains only about 120 calories.

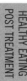

HEALTHY EATING
POST TREATMENT

Eggplant Parmesan 🥕

A quick and easy version of this popular dish.

MAKES 4 TO 5 SERVINGS

2 medium eggplants, peeled and cut in 1/2-inch
   slices (12 slices)
2 onions, sliced into rings
1 (28-ounce) can whole peeled tomatoes,
   undrained
1 teaspoon dried oregano leaves
1/2 teaspoon dried basil leaves
Salt and pepper to taste
1 (8-ounce) package part skim mozzarella cheese,
   shredded

Preheat oven to 350 degrees. Broil eggplant slices 5 inches from heat, about 5 minutes or until brown on one side. Arrange slices, brown side down, in a 2-quart long casserole dish coated with nonstick cooking spray. Top with onions. In a food processor, combine tomatoes with juice, oregano, basil, and salt and pepper, chopping into small pieces. Pour over eggplant. Bake for 45 minutes. Top with mozzarella cheese and bake an additional 15 minutes.

Nutritional information per serving

Calories 230, Protein (g) 16, Carbohydrate (g) 28, Fat (g) 8, Cal. from Fat (%) 29, Saturated Fat (g) 5, Dietary Fiber (g) 9, Cholesterol (mg) 26, Sodium (mg) 455, Diabetic Exchanges: 1.5 lean meat, 6 vegetable

DOC'S NOTES:

Eggplant is very filling, supplying few calories, high in fiber and virtually no fat.

Southwestern Chicken with Salsa ❄

This dish is quick and the homemade salsa baked with the chicken really adds a fabulous something extra. For the salsa, I chop my tomatoes in the food processor.

MAKES 6 SERVINGS

1³/4 pounds boneless skinless chicken breasts
2 teaspoons ground cumin
Salsa (recipe follows)
²/3 cup shredded reduced-fat Monterey
  Jack cheese

Preheat oven to 350 degrees. Coat the chicken breasts on both sides with the cumin. In a large skillet coated with non-stick cooking spray, sauté the breasts over medium heat until brown on both sides. Add salsa and transfer to a baking dish and bake for 20 minutes or until chicken is tender. Sprinkle with the shredded cheese and continue baking until the cheese is melted, about 5 minutes.

SALSA

2 medium tomatoes, chopped
2 tablespoons chopped fresh cilantro
1 tablespoon lime juice
1 teaspoon chopped jalapeño, optional
¹/3 cup chopped onion

Combine the tomato, cilantro, lime juice, jalapeño, and onion in a small bowl.

Nutritional information per serving

Calories 197, Protein (g) 35, Carbohydrate (g) 3, Fat (g) 4, Cal. from Fat (%) 20, Saturated Fat (g) 2, Dietary Fiber (g) 1, Cholesterol (mg) 84, Sodium (mg) 171, Diabetic Exchanges: 4 very lean meat, 1 vegetable

DOC'S NOTES:

Add black beans and corn for added fiber and nutrition.

Chicken with Bean Sauce ❄

Here's a great way to include beans in your meals as the beans dissolve into the sauce and enhance the flavor.

MAKES 6 SERVINGS

2 pounds boneless skinless chicken breasts
1 (16-ounce) can fat-free refried beans
½ cup chopped red onion
2 (10-ounce) cans diced tomatoes and green chiles with their juice
1 cup shredded reduced-fat sharp Cheddar cheese, optional
¼ cup chopped green onions (scallions), optional

Preheat oven to 350 degrees. Place chicken breasts in a 2-quart oblong baking dish coated with nonstick cooking spray. Spread the beans to cover the top of the chicken. Sprinkle with the red onion. Pour the tomatoes and juice evenly over the top. Cover with foil and bake 1 hour 20 minutes or until the chicken is done. Sprinkle with the Cheddar cheese and green onions and serve.

Nutritional information per serving
Calories 247, Protein (g) 39, Carbohydrate (g) 16, Fat (g) 2, Cal. from Fat (%) 7, Saturated Fat (g) 1, Dietary Fiber (g) 5, Cholesterol (mg) 88, Sodium (mg) 770, Diabetic Exchanges: 5 very lean meat, 1 starch, 1 vegetable

DOC'S NOTES:

Substitute diced tomatoes for a less spicy version. Beans are high in fiber, protein, and carbohydrates.

Quick Herb Chicken ✳

I bought a mixed pack of fresh herbs at the grocery and prepared this dish. A mixture of basil, oregano, and rosemary works well. You can always use about 2 teaspoons dry herbs of your choice.

Makes 6 servings

2 tablespoons lemon juice

Black pepper to taste

1 tablespoon minced garlic

2 pounds boneless skinless chicken breasts

1 cup all-purpose flour

2 tablespoons olive oil

2 cups canned fat-free chicken broth

2 tablespoons Dijon mustard

¼ cup fresh herbs, chopped

In a small bowl, mix the lemon juice, pepper, and garlic together to season the chicken. Dredge each piece of seasoned chicken in flour and place in a heated large skillet coated with nonstick cooking spray and olive oil. Brown chicken on each side. In a small bowl, combine broth, mustard, and herbs; add to chicken in pan. Bring to a boil, lower heat, cover and cook until chicken is tender, about 15 to 20 minutes.

Nutritional information per serving

Calories 298, Protein (g) 38, Carbohydrate (g) 18, Fat (g) 7, Cal. from Fat (%) 21, Saturated Fat (g) 1, Dietary Fiber (g) 1, Cholesterol (mg) 88, Sodium (mg) 426, Diabetic Exchanges: 4 very lean meat, 1 starch, 1 fat

DOC'S NOTES:

Pasta tossed with olive oil makes a great side dish.

Chicken Primavera ❄

This is one of my all time favorite chicken pasta recipes. Adjust the onion and garlic to your taste buds.

MAKES 6 TO 8 SERVINGS

1 (12-ounce) package linguine
1½ pounds boneless skinless chicken pieces
¼ cup olive oil
3 cloves garlic, minced
½ pound mushrooms, sliced
1 onion, chopped
1 red bell pepper, cored and chopped
½ teaspoon dried oregano leaves
½ teaspoon dried basil leaves
½ teaspoon dried thyme leaves
Salt and pepper to taste
1 cup frozen peas
¼ cup grated Parmesan cheese

Cook linguine according to directions on package; drain. In a large frying pan, cook chicken pieces in olive oil and garlic until lightly browned and done. Watch carefully, tossing to keep from sticking. Add mushrooms, onions, red pepper, and seasonings, sautéing until tender. Add peas, tossing until heated. When pasta is ready, add to chicken mixture, combining well. Add Parmesan cheese and serve.

Nutritional information per serving
Calories 360, Protein (g) 29, Carbohydrate (g) 39, Fat (g) 10, Cal. from Fat (%) 24, Saturated Fat (g) 2, Dietary Fiber (g) 3, Cholesterol (mg) 52, Sodium (mg) 139, Diabetic Exchanges: 3 lean meat, 2 starch, 1.5 vegetable

DOC'S NOTES:

A quick recipe that will appeal to the family.

Shrimp, Peppers, and Cheese Grits

A nice change is to use grits, which has similar nutritional value to other enriched grains.

MAKES 4 TO 6 SERVINGS

1 green bell pepper, cored and sliced
1/2 cup chopped tomatoes
1 1/2 pounds medium shrimp, peeled
1/2 cup chopped green onions (scallions)
2 cups canned fat-free chicken broth
1 1/2 cups skim milk
1 cup quick grits
1 cup shredded reduced-fat Cheddar cheese

In a large skillet coated with nonstick cooking spray, sauté the green pepper, tomatoes, and shrimp, cooking until the shrimp are done, about 5 to 7 minutes. Add the green onions, cooking several more minutes. Meanwhile, in a pot, bring the chicken broth and milk to a boil. Stir in the grits. Return to a boil, cover, and reduce to low heat. Cook about 5 minutes or until thickened, stir occasionally. Stir in the cheese. Serve the shrimp over the cheese grits.

Nutritional information per serving
Calories 256, Protein (g) 25, Carbohydrate (g) 27, Fat (g) 5, Cal. from Fat (%) 17, Saturated Fat (g) 3, Dietary Fiber (g) 1, Cholesterol (mg) 146, Sodium (mg) 516, Diabetic Exchanges: 3 very lean meat, 1.5 starch, 1 vegetable

DOC'S NOTES:

You have to try this to see how delicious it really is. A great source of Vitamin A and fiber, yet low in fat.

Herbed Shrimp

A quick recipe to enjoy shrimp. Serve with French bread to dip in the sauce. Try serving with sautéed kale—a cruciferous veggie.

MAKES 4 SERVINGS

3/4 cup Worcestershire sauce
3 tablespoons olive oil
2 tablespoons dried rosemary leaves
3 bay leaves
1/3 cup sherry, optional
2 tablespoons lemon juice
1 1/2 pounds large unpeeled shrimp

In a large bowl, combine all ingredients except shrimp. Add shrimp to mixture and marinate in refrigerator at least 2 to 3 hours. Preheat oven to 400 degrees. Transfer shrimp and marinade to an oblong dish and bake for 20 minutes. Watch closely and turn shrimp.

Nutritional information per serving

Calories 234, Protein (g) 22, Carbohydrate (g) 10, Fat (g) 12, Cal. from Fat (%) 45, Saturated Fat (g) 2, Dietary Fiber (g) 1, Cholesterol (mg) 202, Sodium (mg) 733, Diabetic Exchanges: 3 lean meat, 0.5 other carb., 1.5 fat

Baked Topped Fish

Here's a simple and delicious fish recipe.

MAKES 4 SERVINGS

3 tablespoons light mayonnaise
1 tablespoon Worcestershire sauce
1/4 cup chopped green onions (scallions), optional
1/4 teaspoon hot pepper sauce
2 pounds trout fillets or fish of choice
Salt and pepper to taste
2 tablespoons balsamic vinegar

Preheat broiler. In a bowl, combine the mayonnaise, Worcestershire sauce, green onions, and hot sauce. Lay the fillets in a baking dish. Sprinkle with salt and pepper. Spread the mayonnaise mixture evenly over the fillets. Drizzle with the vinegar. Place under the broiler for 6 to 10 minutes or until the fish flakes easily with a fork. Watch carefully so it doesn't burn.

Nutritional information per serving

Calories 379, Protein (g) 47, Carbohydrate (g) 3, Fat (g) 19, Cal. from Fat (%) 45, Saturated Fat (g) 3, Dietary Fiber (g) 0, Cholesterol (mg) 133, Sodium (mg) 252, Diabetic Exchanges: 6 lean meat

DOC'S NOTES:

This is a nice change from red meat. Shrimp are low in fat and calories.

DOC'S NOTES:

Fish is rich in protein, iron, B vitamins, and other nutrients.

Salmon Patties with Horseradish Caper Sauce ❄

If you enjoy salmon, this easy recipe will quickly become a favorite. Perfect when you need a light quick meal. Serve with Horseradish Caper Sauce, over fresh sautéed spinach, or on a whole wheat bun for a great sandwich.

MAKES 6 PATTIES

1¼ pounds salmon fillets, skinned
⅓ cup finely chopped onion
3 tablespoons light mayonnaise
½ teaspoon dried tarragon or dill weed leaves
½ cup Italian bread crumbs
Salt and pepper to taste

Trim salmon and cut into 2-inch cubes; place in the food processor or chop finely by hand. Add the onion, mayonnaise, tarragon, and bread crumbs, mixing well. Season to taste. Coat a skillet with nonstick cooking spray and heat. Make the salmon mixture into six patties and brown the patties over a medium-high heat for 1 minute. Lower heat and continue cooking for a few minutes; turn over and continue cooking about 3 more minutes. Do not overcook. Serve with Horseradish Caper Sauce.

HORSERADISH CAPER SAUCE

¼ cup light mayonnaise
2 tablespoons prepared horseradish
1 tablespoon lemon juice
1 tablespoon finely chopped onion
1 teaspoon capers, drained

Stir all ingredients together and refrigerate.

Nutritional information per serving
Calories 212, Protein (g) 21, Carbohydrate (g) 10, Fat (g) 9, Cal. from Fat (%) 40, Saturated Fat (g) 2, Dietary Fiber (g) 1, Cholesterol (mg) 55, Sodium (mg) 380, Diabetic Exchanges: 3 lean meat, 0.5 starch

DOC'S NOTES:

Salmon is a rich source of omega-3s.

Simply Salmon Pasta

An elegant blend of ingredients and flavors. Salmon contains lots of omega-3 fatty acids, which are being studied for their many possible healthy benefits.

MAKES 6 TO 8 SERVINGS

1 (9-ounce) package spinach tortellini
1 (12 ounce) package bow tie pasta
8 ounces salmon filets
Salt and pepper to taste
1/4 teaspoon sugar
1 cup canned fat-free chicken broth
2/3 cup evaporated skimmed milk
1 cup sugar snap peas
1/2 cup chopped green onions (scallions)
1 teaspoon dried dill weed leaves
1/3 cup grated Parmesan cheese

In a large pot of boiling water, add the spinach tortellini and cook for about 10 minutes. To the same pot, add the bow tie pasta and continue cooking until pasta is done. Drain and set aside. Season the salmon with salt and pepper and sugar. In a skillet coated with nonstick cooking spray, cook the salmon, skin side down, over medium-high heat. Turn to other side and cook until done. Remove skin, cut meat into chunks, and set aside. In the same skillet, add chicken broth and evaporated milk. Bring to a boil, reduce heat, and simmer until liquid reduces, about 7 minutes. Add the peas and green onions, cooking several minutes or until peas are crisp tender. Add the cooked pasta, dill, and cheese, tossing carefully. Carefully toss in the salmon.

Nutritional information per serving
Calories 298, Protein (g) 18, Carbohydrate (g) 43, Fat (g) 5, Cal. from Fat (%) 16, Saturated Fat (g) 2, Dietary Fiber (g) 2, Cholesterol (mg) 60, Sodium (mg) 269, Diabetic Exchanges: 1 lean meat, 3 starch

DOC'S NOTES:

Good source of omegas, iron, calcium and vitamin C.

Herb Baked Salmon

A gourmet delight with little or no effort. Spinach or Swiss chard makes a nice nutritional side.

MAKES 6 SERVINGS

2 pounds salmon fillets
1 tablespoon margarine, melted
Salt and pepper to taste
1 tablespoon finely chopped parsley
1/4 cup Dijon honey mustard
1/4 teaspoon dried thyme leaves
1/2 teaspoon minced garlic
1/4 teaspoon dried marjoram, optional
1/4 teaspoon dried rosemary leaves
1 tablespoon lemon juice

Preheat oven to 350 degrees. Place salmon fillets in an oblong baking dish coated with nonstick cooking spray. In a bowl combine melted margarine, salt and pepper, parsley, mustard, thyme, garlic, marjoram, rosemary, and lemon juice. Pour mixture over salmon. Cover with foil. Bake for 30 to 35 minutes or grill if desired. Serve with veggies.

Nutritional information per serving

Calories 214, Protein (g) 30, Carbohydrate (g) 4, Fat (g) 7, Cal. from Fat (%) 32, Saturated Fat (g) 1, Dietary Fiber (g) 0, Cholesterol (mg) 79, Sodium (mg) 134, Diabetic Exchanges: 4 lean meat

DOC'S NOTES:

Salmon contains omega 3 fatty acids. Omega 3's have anti-clotting properties and may be protective against heart attacks and perhaps high blood pressure.

Tuna Steaks with Horseradish Sauce

Marinate the steaks, cook, and serve with this incredible sauce for an effortless, outstanding meal. "The easy gourmet!" The tuna may also be grilled or cooked inside on a grill skillet. Tuna is high in protein and low in fat.

MAKES 4 SERVINGS

4 (6- to 8-ounce) tuna steaks or fillets
1/2 cup teriyaki sauce
1/2 cup fat-free Italian dressing
1/2 cup nonfat plain yogurt
1/2 tablespoon prepared horseradish
1 tablespoon Dijon mustard

Rinse the tuna steaks and pat dry. In a flat dish, combine the teriyaki sauce and Italian dressing with the tuna. Cover and refrigerate for at least 2 hours. Heat a skillet coated with nonstick cooking spray over medium heat until hot. Cook the tuna about 3 to 5 minutes on each side, depending on thickness, until done. In a small bowl, mix together the yogurt, horseradish, and mustard. Top each steak with a dollop of sauce before serving.

Nutritional information per serving

*Calories 218, Protein (g) 42, Carbohydrate (g) 5,
Fat (g) 2, Cal. from Fat (%) 8, Saturated Fat (g) 1,
Dietary Fiber (g) 0, Cholesterol (mg) 77, Sodium (mg) 595,
Diabetic Exchanges: 5 very lean meat, 0.5 other carb.*

DOC'S NOTES:

Tuna is a fish rich in omega 3 fatty acids.

Meaty Cabbage Casserole ❄

This recipe is a quick and easy alternative to individually stuffing all those cabbage leaves; yet has the same appeal.

MAKES 6 TO 8 SERVINGS

1½ pounds ground sirloin
1 onion chopped
1 teaspoon minced garlic
¼ teaspoon black pepper
3 cups cooked white or brown rice
1 (¾-pound) head of cabbage, coarsely shredded
1 (27-ounce) jar spaghetti sauce
¼ cup light brown sugar
1 cup shredded reduced-fat Cheddar cheese

Preheat oven to 350 degrees. In a large skillet, cook the beef, onion, and garlic until the beef is done. Drain any excess grease. Add the pepper and cooked rice, mixing well. Spoon the meat mixture into a 3-quart casserole dish coated with nonstick cooking spray. Top with the shredded cabbage. In a bowl, mix together the spaghetti sauce and brown sugar. Pour the sauce over the cabbage. Bake, covered, for 1 hour, 15 minutes, or until the cabbage is tender. Sprinkle with the Cheddar cheese and continue baking for 5 minutes, or until the cheese is melted.

Nutritional information per serving
Calories 366, Protein (g) 25, Carbohydrate (g) 38, Fat (g) 12, Cal. from Fat (%) 30, Saturated Fat (g) 5, Dietary Fiber (g) 3, Cholesterol (mg) 39, Sodium (mg) 619, Diabetic Exchanges: 3 lean meat, 1 starch, 3 vegetable, 0.5 other carb.

DOC'S NOTES:

Cabbage is a cruciferous vegetable which has been identified as possibly being protective against cancer.

Italian-Style Pot Roast ❄

This well-flavored recipe can also be made in a slow cooker. Everyone loves a pot roast and gravy. Serve this with rice or potatoes.

MAKES 8 TO 10 SERVINGS

1 (4- to 5-pound) beef round roast

2 cups canned beef broth

1/2 cup Burgundy wine, optional

3 tablespoons no-salt-added tomato paste

1 (28-ounce) can no-salt-added whole tomatoes, chopped, with their juice

2 cloves garlic, minced

1 tablespoon dried basil leaves

1 tablespoon dried oregano leaves

2 bay leaves

1 pound carrots, cut into 1-inch pieces

3 onions quartered

1 pound fresh mushrooms, halved

1 tablespoon margarine

2 tablespoons all-purpose flour

Preheat oven to 350 degrees. Place the roast in a large pot. Pour in the beef broth and wine. Add the tomato paste and stir. Add the tomatoes with their juice. Blend in the garlic, basil, oregano, and bay leaves. Cover and cook in the oven for 1 1/2 hours. Add the carrots, onions, and mushrooms. Cover and continue cooking for 1 1/2 hours or until the meat is tender. Transfer the meat to a carving board. Mash the margarine and flour together to form a paste. Place the pot over medium high heat and bring the liquid to a boil. Whisk in the paste to thicken the sauce. Serve meat with the vegetables and the sauce. Discard bay leaves.

Nutritional information per serving

Calories 399, Protein (g) 54, Carbohydrate (g) 17, Fat (g) 11, Cal. from Fat (%) 26, Saturated Fat (g) 4, Dietary Fiber (g) 4, Cholesterol (mg) 123, Sodium (mg) 366, Diabetic Exchanges: 6 lean meat, 3 vegetable

DOCTOR'S NOTES:

Good source of vitamin A, B, and protein.

Grilled Pork Tenderloin ❄

Pork tenderloins are very lean and a great alternative to chicken or beef. Keep tenderloins in your freezer to defrost for a quick dinner.

MAKES 6 SERVINGS

1 teaspoon olive oil
¼ cup balsamic vinegar
1 tablespoon honey
1 teaspoon Dijon mustard
1 teaspoon dried rosemary leaves
2 (1-pound) pork tenderloins

In a small bowl, combine the olive oil, balsamic vinegar, honey, Dijon mustard, and rosemary. Trim the fat from the tenderloins. Place tenderloins in a dish and pour the marinade over them. Refrigerate for 2 hours or longer. Preheat oven to 350 degrees. Place the tenderloins on a rack in a roasting pan coated with nonstick cooking spray. Bake for 50 minutes to 1 hour or until a meat thermometer registers 160 degrees. Baste frequently with the marinade and discard any remaining after cooking.

Nutritional information per serving
Calories 200, Protein (g) 32, Carbohydrate (g) 3,
Fat (g) 6, Cal. from Fat (%) 28, Saturated Fat (g) 2,
Dietary Fiber (g) 0, Cholesterol (mg) 90, Sodium (mg) 75,
Diabetic Exchanges: 4 lean meat

DOC'S NOTES:

Easy source of protein.

Savory Lamb Chops ❄

Rich in flavor, these chops will please any palate. I even use this marinade with veal and beef. Serve with veggies and a baked sweet potato for a complete meal.

MAKES 6 TO 8 SERVINGS

1 cup canned beef broth
3 tablespoons orange marmalade
3 tablespoons balsamic vinegar
1/4 cup chopped onion
1 tablespoon dried marjoram
1 tablespoon dried rosemary leaves
1 tablespoon minced garlic
2 pounds lamb loin chops (1-inch thick), excess fat trimmed

In a shallow dish, combine beef broth, marmalade, vinegar, onion, marjoram, rosemary, and garlic. Pour the marinade over lamb chops. Cover and marinate in refrigerator 8 hours or overnight, turning occasionally. Preheat grill to medium or turn on broiler. Grill or broil lamb 8 to 15 minutes on each side or to desired doneness, basting with reserved marinade. Discard any leftover marinade.

Nutritional information per serving

Calories 123, Protein (g) 15, Carbohydrate (g) 3, Fat (g) 5, Cal. from Fat (%) 37, Saturated Fat (g) 2, Dietary Fiber (g) 0, Cholesterol (mg) 48, Sodium (mg) 108, Diabetic Exchanges: 2 lean meat

DOC'S NOTES:

Lamb is leaner than most cuts of beef. It is an excellent source of protein, iron, zinc, and Vitamin B12.

Italian Veal Supreme ❄

Veal and pasta are a natural together, and with the spices and olives, this dish has a distinct personality. There is not a lot of sauce in this dish but there is a lot of flavor.

MAKES 6 SERVINGS

1 (12-ounce) package angel hair pasta

1 large onion, thinly sliced

1 pound thinly sliced veal (scaloppini),
   cut into 1-inch strips

2 tablespoons all-purpose flour

1/2 cup dry white wine or chicken broth

1 teaspoon minced garlic

Salt and pepper to taste

1 teaspoon dried oregano leaves

1 teaspoon dried thyme leaves

5 medium plum (Roma) tomatoes,
   cut into wedges

1 (2¼-ounce) can sliced ripe black
   olives, drained

2 tablespoons chopped parsley

Cook the pasta according to package directions; drain and set aside. In a large skillet coated with nonstick cooking spray, over medium heat, sauté the onion until tender, about 5 minutes. Sprinkle the veal with the flour and add the veal to the skillet, stirring constantly, cooking the veal until lightly browned. Stir in the wine, garlic, salt and pepper, oregano, and thyme. Bring to a boil; cover, reduce the heat, and simmer 8 to 10 minutes or until the veal is almost tender. Add the tomatoes and olives; cover and simmer 5 minutes or until thoroughly heated. Serve the veal mixture over the pasta; sprinkle with parsley.

Nutritional information per serving

Calories 354, Protein (g) 25, Carbohydrate (g) 51, Fat (g) 4, Cal. from Fat (%) 9, Saturated Fat (g) 1, Dietary Fiber (g) 3, Cholesterol (mg) 59, Sodium (mg) 153, Diabetic Exchanges: 2 very lean meat, 3 starch, 1 vegetable

DOC'S NOTES:

Good source of vitamin A and protein.

Almost Better
Than Sex Cake ✎ ❄

The name says it all when you have a sweet tooth and this is such an easy recipe. Keep ingredients in pantry to prepare anytime.

MAKES 20 SERVINGS

1 (18¼-ounce) box yellow cake mix
½ cup skim milk
¼ cup water
⅓ cup canola oil
2 large eggs
2 large egg whites
1 cup nonfat plain yogurt
1 (4-serving) box instant vanilla pudding
1 (4-ounce) bar German chocolate, grated
⅓ cup semi-sweet chocolate chips
½ cup chopped pecans

Preheat oven to 350 degrees. Combine all ingredients except chocolate chips and pecans in a large mixing bowl. Beat slightly, only until mixture is combined. Stir in chocolate chips and pecans. Pour batter into a 10-inch fluted Bundt pan coated with nonstick cooking spray and dusted with flour. Bake for 50 to 55 minutes. Do not overbake.

Nutritional information per serving
Calories 240, Protein (g) 4, Carbohydrate (g) 32,
Fat (g) 12, Cal. from Fat (%) 43, Saturated Fat (g) 2,
Dietary Fiber (g) 1, Cholesterol (mg) 22, Sodium (mg) 263,
Diabetic Exchanges: 2 other carb., 2.5 fat

DOC'S NOTES:

Chocolate is an antioxidant!

Banana Cake with Cream Cheese Icing ✐ ❄

Try using 1 1/2 cups whole wheat flour and 1 cup all-purpose flour. For a variation add 1/2 cup mini chocolate chips or golden raisins. When you have ripe bananas, it's time for this cake.

MAKES 16 TO 20 SERVINGS

2 1/2 cups all-purpose flour
1 teaspoon baking powder
1 1/2 teaspoons baking soda
1 teaspoon ground cinnamon
1/4 cup canola oil
1 cup dark brown sugar
2 large eggs
1 1/2 cups mashed bananas
2 teaspoons vanilla extract
1 cup buttermilk

Preheat oven to 350 degrees. In a bowl, combine flour, baking powder, baking soda, and cinnamon; set aside. In a mixing bowl, beat oil and brown sugar until light. Add eggs, mixing well. Add bananas and vanilla. Add dry ingredients alternately with buttermilk. Pour batter evenly into three 9-inch round baking pans coated with nonstick cooking spray. Bake for 20 minutes or until a toothpick inserted comes out clean. Cool and ice.

CREAM CHEESE ICING

1 (8-ounce) package light cream cheese, softened
3 tablespoons margarine, softened
1 (16-ounce) box confectioners' sugar
1 teaspoon vanilla extract

In a mixing bowl, beat the cream cheese and margarine until smooth. Add the confectioners' sugar and beat until light. Blend in the vanilla. When cake is cool, ice with Cream Cheese Icing.

Nutritional information per serving
Calories 284, Protein (g) 4, Carbohydrate (g) 50, Fat (g) 8, Cal. from Fat (%) 24, Saturated Fat (g) 2, Dietary Fiber (g) 1, Cholesterol (mg) 30, Sodium (mg) 207, Diabetic Exchanges: 0.5 fruit, 3 other carb., 1.5 fat

Strawberry Angel Food Cake 🥕

Great during strawberry season as it's so light and so quick! Buy an angel food cake at the grocery or you can prepare a mix.

MAKES 10 TO 12 SLICES

1 (16-ounce) commercially prepared angel food cake
1 (8-ounce) package light cream cheese, softened
½ cup sugar
¼ cup evaporated skimmed milk
2 pints strawberries, hulled and sliced

Use a serrated knife to slice the angel food cake horizontally into 3 equal layers. Prepare the filling by creaming together the cream cheese, sugar, and evaporated skimmed milk. Top the bottom cake layer with the filling and strawberries. Repeat the layers. Refrigerate.

Nutritional information per serving

Calories 190, Protein (g) 5, Carbohydrate (g) 35, Fat (g) 3, Cal. from Fat (%) 16, Saturated Fat (g) 2, Dietary Fiber (g) 2, Cholesterol (mg) 9, Sodium (mg) 378, Diabetic Exchanges: 0.5 fruit, 2 other carb., 0.5 fat

DOC'S NOTES:

What a great way to enjoy getting vitamin C, potassium and ellagic acid.

Peanut Butter Banana Pie 🥕

Firm bananas rather than extra-ripe ones work best in this pie.

MAKES 8 SERVINGS

1¼ cups reduced-fat vanilla wafer crumbs
  (about 30 cookies)
2 tablespoons margarine, melted
²⁄₃ cup sugar
3 tablespoons cornstarch
1½ cups skim milk
2 eggs, lightly beaten
2 tablespoons reduced-fat crunchy peanut butter
1 teaspoon vanilla extract
3 cups sliced banana
1½ cups frozen fat-free whipped topping, thawed

In a small bowl, mix together the vanilla wafer crumbs and margarine. Press into a 9-inch pie plate; set aside. Combine sugar and cornstarch in a small heavy saucepan. Gradually add milk, stirring with a whisk until well-blended. Cook over medium heat until mixture comes to a boil. Cook for 1 minute, stirring with a whisk. Gradually add about ⅓ cup hot custard to beaten eggs, stirring constantly with a whisk. Return egg mixture to saucepan. Cook over medium heat, stirring constantly, for about 1 minute or until thick. Remove from heat and stir in peanut butter and vanilla. Cool slightly. Arrange banana slices in bottom of prepared crust; spoon filling over bananas. Press plastic wrap onto the surface of filling; refrigerate until well chilled. Remove plastic wrap. Spread whipped topping evenly over filling. Refrigerate.

Nutritional information per serving

Calories 288, Protein (g) 5, Carbohydrate (g) 52, Fat (g) 7, Cal. from Fat (%) 21, Saturated Fat (g) 1, Dietary Fiber (g) 2, Cholesterol (mg) 54, Sodium (mg) 153,

DOC'S NOTES:

Bananas are a great source of potassium, while peanut butter is a great source of protein, iron, magnesium, and fiber. Potassium is vital for muscle contraction, nerve impulses, and proper function of the heart and kidneys.

Ambrosia Crumble

For this recipe, I suggest using fresh fruit, and for a real treat, serve over frozen vanilla yogurt. This is one of those desserts I attack right when it comes out of the oven.

MAKES 10 SERVINGS

1 cup all-purpose flour
1/2 cup light brown sugar
3 tablespoons margarine
1/4 cup flaked coconut
2 cups fresh pineapple chunks
3 large navel oranges, peeled and sectioned
3 large bananas, cut into 1/2-inch thick slices
2 tablespoons lemon juice
1 teaspoon coconut extract

Preheat oven to 350 degrees. In a bowl, combine the flour and brown sugar; cut in the margarine with a pastry blender or fork until the mixture is crumbly. Set aside. In a bowl, combine the coconut, pineapple, oranges, bananas, lemon juice, and coconut extract; toss well. Place the fruit mixture in a 13×9×2-inch baking dish coated with nonstick cooking spray. Sprinkle with the reserved flour mixture. Bake, uncovered, for 45 minutes, until golden.

Nutritional information per serving

Calories 206, Protein (g) 3, Carbohydrate (g) 40, Fat (g) 5, Cal. from Fat (%) 20, Saturated Fat (g) 2, Dietary Fiber (g) 3, Cholesterol (mg) 0, Sodium (mg) 55, Diabetic Exchanges: 0.5 starch, 1 fruit, 1 other carb., 1 fat

DOC'S NOTES:

Excellent source of Vitamin C and potassium.

Index